A.I. Shvets
A. S. Nekhlopochin
A. A. Baranishin

Spinal cord trauma in X-ray, CT and MRI studies

A.I. Shvets
A. S. Nekhlopochin
A. A. Baranishin

Spinal cord trauma in X-ray, CT and MRI studies

to help the practicing physician

ScienciaScripts

Imprint
Any brand names and product names mentioned in this book are subject to trademark, brand or patent protection and are trademarks or registered trademarks of their respective holders. The use of brand names, product names, common names, trade names, product descriptions etc. even without a particular marking in this work is in no way to be construed to mean that such names may be regarded as unrestricted in respect of trademark and brand protection legislation and could thus be used by anyone.

Cover image: www.ingimage.com

This book is a translation from the original published under ISBN 978-620-2-06751-5.

Publisher:
Sciencia Scripts
is a trademark of
Dodo Books Indian Ocean Ltd. and OmniScriptum S.R.L publishing group

120 High Road, East Finchley, London, N2 9ED, United Kingdom
Str. Armeneasca 28/1, office 1, Chisinau MD-2012, Republic of Moldova, Europe
Printed at: see last page
ISBN: 978-620-7-93962-6

Table of contents

Authors

Shvets Alexey Ivanovich - Doctor of Medical Sciences, Professor of the Department of
Traumatology and Orthopedics.
Lugansk
State Medical
University. Lugansk city.

Nekhlopochin Oleksii Sergeevich - resident, Akad. A.P. Romodanov Research Institute of Neurosurgery, Kiev.

Nekhlopochin Sergey Nikolaevich - Candidate of Medical Sciences, Lugansk Republican Clinical Hospital, Lugansk, Russia

Baranishin Oleksandr Anatolievich - radiologist, Omega-Kyiv DMC, Kyiv.

The severity of spinal injuries and sometimes irreversible changes in the spine, a large percentage of disability among young and able-bodied people determine the social significance of solving the complex problem of diagnosis, treatment and rehabilitation of these patients, as well as the prevention of spinal cord and spinal cord injuries.

The authors of the monograph based on their own clinical experience and literature data highlighted modern approaches and views on the diagnosis of the most common spinal injuries in clinical practice.

The material includes illustrations in the form of drawings and photocopies of radiographs, CT, MRI, which clearly show the picture of the injury and are accompanied by explanations of the features of the image and the correspondence of images on radiographs, CT and MRI to the classifications of spinal injuries.

The monograph is presented as a manual to assist the practical physician for traumatologists, neurosurgeons and surgeons, as well as interns of the relevant profile.

Spinal cord injury in X-ray, CT and MRI studies

INTRODUCTION

Spinal cord injuries are characterized by great diversity in the nature and extent of damage, represent one of the most complex sections of traumatology and remain an important medical and social problem. Urbanization and the development of society, constantly improving industrialization, motorization and the growth of floor space in cities and districts contribute to a high proportion of spinal injuries and their severity. In a significant number of cases, spinal trauma is accompanied by a violation of the integrity and shape of the vertebral body and adjacent discs, spinal canal, violation of physiological curves and formation of kyphosis.

According to different authors, spinal injuries occur in 3.1 to 9% of all musculoskeletal injuries. In terms of damage localization, the first place is occupied by the lumbo-thoracic and lumbar spine, the second by the thoracic spine, and the third by the cervical spine. Damage to the spinal cord and spinal nerves is diagnosed in 23.8 - 34.5 % of the total number of spinal injuries.

Disability after spinal cord injuries ranks second among all musculoskeletal injuries after tibia fractures (18.7% and 34.5%), respectively. During the initial examination at the MSEC, up to 63.9% of patients with uncomplicated spinal injuries are recognized as disabled. Of these, 0.2% are Group 1 disabled, 65.3% are Group 1 disabled, and 34.5% are Group 6 disabled. Among patients with complicated spinal injuries, about 10% with irreversible changes die at the site of injury, 10% with neurological manifestations after conservative treatment or emergency surgical interventions restore the lost functions of the spinal cord and spine, and the remaining 80%, having gone through all stages of traumatic disease, require complex, long-term rehabilitation measures and remain disabled of groups 1 - P.

The severity of spinal injuries and sometimes irreversible changes in the spine, a large percentage of disability among young and able-bodied people determine the social significance of solving the complex problem of treatment and rehabilitation of these patients, as well as the prevention of spinal cord and spinal cord injuries.

Anatomical features

The spine is a complex anatomical organ that should always be considered in statics and dynamics, i.e. from anatomical and physiological (biomechanical) positions. In addition, it should be remembered that the spine is not only an organ of support and movement, but also a case, a receptacle of the most complex organ - the spinal cord and its elements, and therefore the features of the structure of the spine at all levels and the functions of the spine are closely related to the spinal cord and its elements. The vertebra consists of 24, sometimes 25 individual vertebrae, and includes 7 cervical, 12 thoracic, 5 lumbar vertebrae. Together with the sacrum (4-5 fused sacral vertebrae) and coccyx (4-5 fused coccygeal vertebrae), they form a single column - the vertebral column. In the spine, according to the named vertebrae are distinguished departments: cervical, thoracic, lumbar and sacral. Given the functional and biomechanical features in the areas of transition of the mobile spine to the immobile spine, the so-called transitional sections are distinguished - the thoracolumbar, including two lower thoracic and two upper lumbar vertebrae, cervical-thoracic, lumbosacral.

There are four curvatures in the spinal column in the sagittal plane: cervical lordosis, thoracic kyphosis, lumbar lordosis, and sacral kyphosis. These curvatures are physiological, compensatory in nature, so their magnitudes are always directly proportional to each other (Fig. 1.). If thoracic kyphosis increases for any reason, lumbar lordosis increases and vice versa.

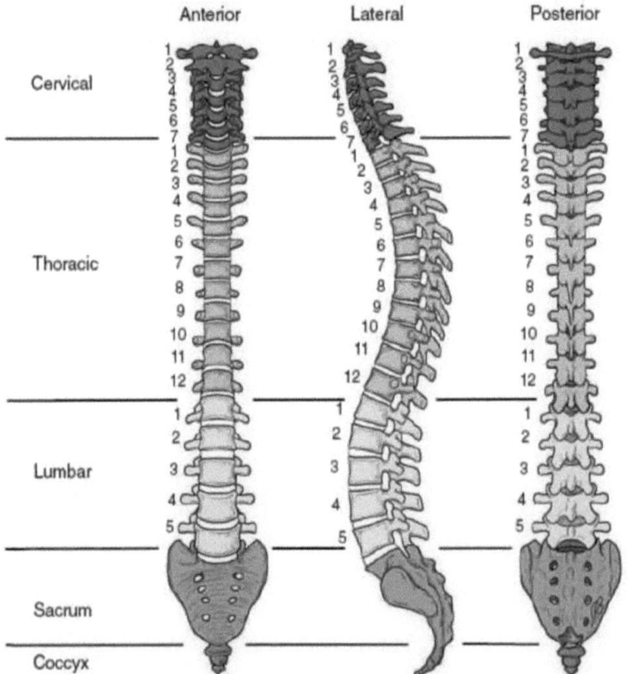

Figure 1. Physiologic curves and anatomical sections of the spine

The anatomical structure of the vertebral column and its topographic and anatomical location affect its X-ray image. Due to the layering of shadows of adjacent organs and skeletal parts, as well as the complexity of the anatomical structure of the vertebra itself, diagnostic errors in spinal injuries are noted in 1225% of cases. This applies primarily to damage to individual vertebral elements and the representation of vertebrae in transitional sections of the spine.

All sections of the spine are characterized by anatomical and topographical features that have a leading role in the function of these sections and are reflected in the features of vertebral injuries in trauma. The two upper cervical vertebrae occupy a special place. Between the occipital bone and the atlantus, as well as between the atlantus and the epistropheum, there is no intervertebral disk that softens and evenly distributes the force during impact. In addition, the atlas has no body and consists of an anterior and posterior wishbone. Its wishbones are thin, easily broken, and the entire vertebra is a ring located between the head and the second cervical vertebra.

First cervical vertebra (atlantis)

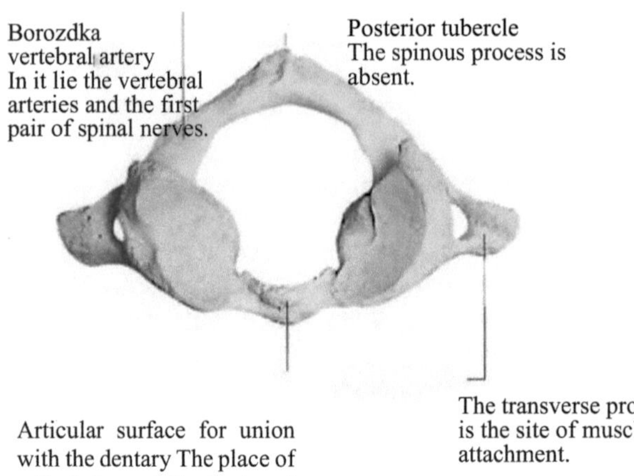

The second cervical vertebra is also distinguished from all other vertebrae by the presence of a tooth. From the front, the tooth articulates with the inner surface of the anterior half of the atlantus to form the Creuvillier joint, while behind it, a strong transverse ligament runs transversely, limiting the tooth's posterior displacement. The other cervical vertebrae are similar to each other in structure and form of articulation and differ fundamentally from the structure of vertebrae in other sections by the saddle-shaped connection of the vertebral bodies with each other, forming Luschka's uncovertebral joints in the lateral sections (Luschka, 1956). The short transverse processes of the cervical vertebrae have round holes (foramina vertebralia) through which the vertebral artery and vein pass. Normally, the vertebral artery enters the opening of the transverse process of the sixth cervical vertebra, rises vertically up to the upper surface of the transverse process of the atlantus and, bending steeply, reaches the posterior atlanto-occipital membrane.

The thoracic spine is the most rigid. The intervertebral discs between the vertebral bodies are low, and all vertebrae are connected to a single rigid framework by means of ribs. The articular processes of the thoracic vertebrae are located in the frontal plane. In the lumbar region, the articular processes are located mainly in the sagittal plane or close to it.

Mechanism of spinal cord injury

The **flexor mechanism** is triggered by a sudden, sudden, one-step forced bending of the torso or head tilt. This mechanism of violence occurs in a fall from a height on the buttocks or on straightened legs, in a rock or soil blockage in a sitting or squatting position. In this mechanism of injury in the thoracic, thoracolumbar spine, compression fractures occur more often. If excessive sharp bending loads continue after the fracture, the violence leads to vertebral dislocation and fracture-dislocation occurs.

The **extensor mechanism of** violence is a much less common cause of injury and is more characteristic of the cervical spine. Characteristic in this case are injuries in car collisions and in divers. In the first case, there is a so-called whiplash movement, when the head is sharply deflected to the rear with a sharp forced extension of the neck followed by a sharp bending.

In divers, the extensor mechanism occurs when the head is extended. In this case, the diver strikes the frontoparietal region against the bottom or a protruding object. For the thoracic and lumbar spine, the extensor mechanism of violence is characteristic only when falling on the back on a protruding solid object (large log, stone, barrel, rail, etc.).

Rotational (rotational) mechanism of injury in its pure form is extremely rare and its effect is distributed to the cervical and lumbar spine. In the cervical region, this mechanism is possible during sports activities in wrestlers, when incorrect or ineptly performed moves with head rotation. In the lumbar region, this mechanism occurs when a person is caught between two moving machines or between a hard surface (wall) and a moving machine. In miners, this injury occurs when a victim is caught between moving cars, a moving underground train and a wall or pillar.

More characteristic is the combined flexion-rotation mechanism of violence that occurs when a weight is dropped on one shoulder or scapula region of a somewhat bent person, when the violence acts asymmetrically, bending and twisting the spine.

Compression (explosive) mechanism of injury.

The traumatic force in this mechanism acts strictly along the vertical axis of the vertebral segments. Such conditions are created when, at the moment of force application in the vertical spine, the cervical or lumbar spine is in a position of moderate flexion, in which the physiologic lordosis is smoothed. The entire force acts in a "straight spine" on the pulposus nucleus, which, being in an enclosed space and having no tendency to compress, transmits all the enormous axial force acting evenly in all directions. With a preserved disc, the fibrous ring withstands these loads, the closure plate of one of the vertebrae along with hyaline cartilage bursts, and the fluid pulposus nucleus rushing with tremendous force into a weak spot breaks the vertebral body into separate fragments according to the law of hydraulic effect. When the posterior fragment is displaced toward the spinal canal, spinal cord contusion, hematomyelia (cerebral hemorrhage) or its crushing is possible. Compression-slip fractures occur. Some authors call such fractures "blast" fractures. In contrast to flexion compression fractures, in which there is compression (compression) of the vertebral body and a decrease in its height, in explosive fractures, the term "compression" includes a mechanism of violence. However, if the bending motion continues after the explosive effect, deformation (compression) of the already destroyed vertebra may occur.

The posterior support complex in blast fractures most often remains intact, and according to the classical Holdworth scheme, these fractures should be classified as stable. However, in the absence of anterior support, the spine cannot be stable, and kyphosis gradually increases with all its consequences.

Shear injuries occur when a force is applied in the horizontal plane and more often in stiff spine regions, when the lower part of the spine has a solid base. Most often such injuries are localized in the thoracic spine, less often in the thoracolumbar and lumbosacral spine. In the cervical spine, in contrast to the flexion mechanism that leads to a tipping dislocation, sharp violence in the anteroposterior direction gives, as defined by Y.L. Tsivyan, a shearing dislocation.

Shear force results in a fracture-dislocation with disruption of anterior and posterior anatomical structures. As a rule, damage to bony structures is accompanied by severe damage to the spinal cord.

Tension injuries: The application of acting forces in a tensile position seems at first glance unnatural and contrary to logic. Nevertheless, in recent years there have been more and more frequent reports of this mechanism of injury in automobile accidents. Inertial movement of the upper half of the torso relative to the fixed lower half is the leading one. This occurs when the torso is fixed with a seat belt. When the upper half of the torso moves by inertia, the lumbar spine is stretched and the intervertebral disc, anterior and posterior longitudinal ligaments, all structures of the posterior ligamentous-summary apparatus and, often, the spinal cord are ruptured. Characteristic of this type of violence is a combined injury, in which, in addition to spinal cord injury, the organs of the abdominal cavity and pelvis, craniocerebral trauma are damaged. In the literature, these injuries are known as seat belt syndrome. In this case, the fracture line may pass through the vertebral body (Chance fracture), through the ligaments and disc, combinations of the 1st and 2nd injuries (Fig. 2).

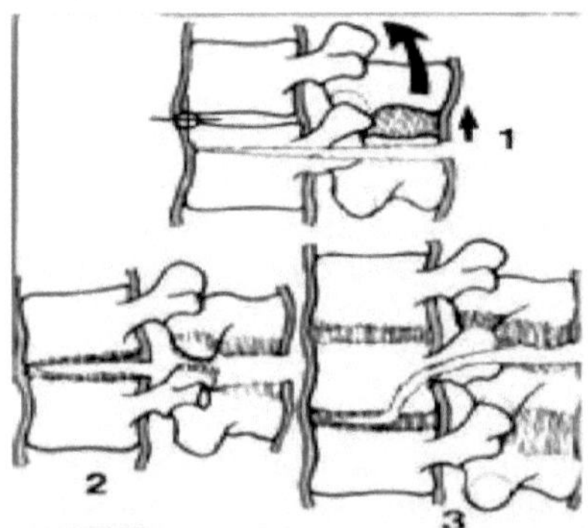

Figure 2. Seat-belt injury type (tether-belt injuries). The fracture line goes through the bone (Chance fracture) (1); - through the ligaments and disk (2), - combination of the first two variants (3).

In addition to the distraction mechanism of injury in car accidents, there is another specific mechanism of injury, the so-called whiplash mechanism, which is characteristic of the cervical spine in car collisions (Fig. 3).

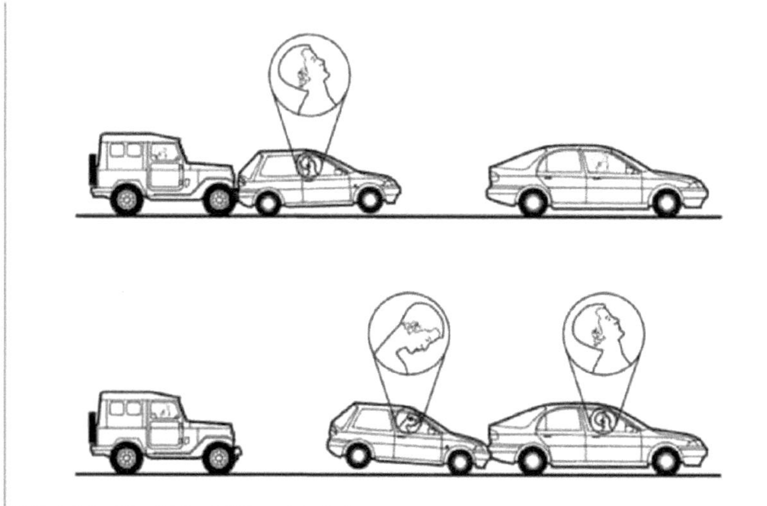

Figure 3. Whiplash mechanism of injury in road trauma

In a rear-end collision, the head of a passenger in a vehicle ahead of the vehicle is first deflected sharply backward (a typical extensor injury), and in the next instant the mechanism of inertial movement is activated and a sharp bending response is triggered, resulting in an additional, already flexor injury. These are the mechanisms that can lead to severe fracture-dislocations with spinal cord injury.

Each of the listed types of violence leads to a certain form of damage to the vertebral column - wedge compression fracture (flexion), dislocation (flexion), disc rupture and damage to posterior structures (extension), splinter fracture, explosive fracture (vertical load). The relationship between the nature of the injury and the mechanism of injury can be conditionally represented as follows.

Classification of injuries by mechanism of trauma origin

Hyperflexion lesions	Hyperextension injuries	Compression injuries	Rotational injuries	Translational damage
Anterior subluxation (hyperflexion distortion)	Hyperextension sprains.	Blast fractures	Rotational subluxations	Fractures of the hook-shaped processes
Hyperflexion dislocations.	Isolated fractures of the C1 vertebral arch	Jefferson fractures	Unilateral intervertebral dislocations	
			joints (+ hyperflexion)	
Tooth fractures	Isolated fractures of the		Colonic fractures	

C2	arch plate		(+hyperextension)	
Wedge fractures of vertebral bodies	The fractures of the "executioner"		Fractures at the border of the stem and arch plate	
Chance fractures	Extension injuries with tear-shaped fragment detachment			
Bilateral dislocations in the intervertebral joints				
Flexion injuries with tear-shaped fragment detachment				
Digger fractures				

There may be combinations of these mechanisms of violence. Head-down falls are most dangerous for the cervical spine. This includes so-called diver's fracture-dislocations, a typical summertime injury. The extensor mechanism is more characteristic. When diving, the victim hits the frontal surface of the head against the bottom or an obstacle. The presence of wounds or abrasions in the frontoparietal region confirm this mechanism and should alert the doctor to the possibility of such an injury.

Classification of spinal injuries

The abuses listed above can lead to injuries that fall into two main categories - stable and unstable.

The concept of stable and unstable spinal fractures was introduced by Nicoli in 1949 for the lumbar spine, and in 1963 Holdworth extended it to the entire spine. The entire spinal column according to Holdworth is divided conventionally into anterior and posterior sections. The posterior spine is formed by all anatomical formations that are located behind the posterior longitudinal ligament. In this case, the arch joints with their ligamentous apparatus, yellow, intercostal and supraspinous ligaments form a complex that Holdworth called the "posterior ligamentous complex", and Y.L. Tsivyan (1971) called the "posterior support complex".

According to this classification, all spinal injuries in which the posterior support complex remains intact are stable. These include, first of all, isolated injuries of individual elements of the posterior complex, first-degree wedge fractures of vertebral bodies without pronounced kyphosis. Moderate anterior injuries are usually not accompanied by damage to the posterior bone and ligamentous structures. In unstable injuries, the posterior support complex is damaged along with the anterior complex. Typical examples of unstable injuries are vertebral dislocations, fracture-dislocations, third-degree compression fractures with a pronounced kyphotic deformity, in which the posterior vertebral elements fan out and the supraspinous and interspinous ligaments are damaged and the joints are subluxed.

To determine the stability of a fracture, the theory of dividing the spine into 3 columns is now more commonly used (Denis F., 1984). According to this theory, the spinal column is divided into three columns: 1 - anterior, which is formed by the anterior longitudinal ligament, the anterior half of the vertebral body, and the anterior part of the intervertebral disc; 2 - middle, which is formed by the posterior half of the vertebral body, the posterior part of the disc, the posterior longitudinal ligament, and the anterior portions of the vertebral pedicles; 3 - posterior support, which is formed by the vertebral arches, arch joints, spinous processes, and the yellow, interorbital, and supraspinous ligaments (Fig. 4). (In a number of literature sources one can find references to the anterior 2/3 of the vertebral body and posterior 1/3 of the vertebral body).

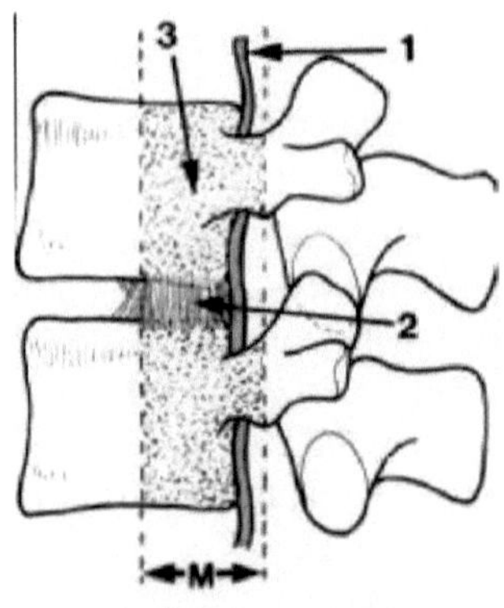

Fig.4 . The three supporting columns of the spine (Denis). Anterior column - up to the vertical dashed line. Middle column (M) - between the two dashed lines. Posterior column - area posterior to the posterior dashed line.

If any two of the listed columns are damaged, the damage is considered unstable.

A three-column model of spinal anatomy.

	Anatomical component	Optimal visualization
Front column	Anterior 2/3 or 1/2 of the vertebral body Anterior 2/3 or 1/2 of the fibrous ring Anterior longitudinal ligament	Sagital front reformats
Center column	Posterior third (or half) of the body and legs of the vertebral arch Posterior third (or half) of the fibrous ring Posterior longitudinal ligament	Axial slices Sagital renormalizations
Rear Column	Posterior part of the arch and articular processes with intervertebral joints Yellow ligaments The supraorbital and interorbital ligaments	Axial slices Sagital and front reformats

Signs of instability after spinal cord injury:

Front column

1. Decrease in body height more than 50%

2. Angular deformity of the vertebral body more than 10%

3. Tear of the anterior longitudinal ligament (tear symptom)

Center column

1. Contour irregularity on the posterior surface of the vertebral body

2.   Decreased height of the vertebral body at the posterior margin

3.   Dislocation of the posterior edge of the vertebral body

4.   Asymmetry of the arch legs or their extension

Rear column

1.   Splitting and divergence of the spinous processes

2.   Fractures extending to the arch pedicles and plate or to the intervertebral joints

3.   Lateral displacement of the articular processes

4.   Subluxation in intervertebral joints with congruence of articular surfaces less than 50%

5.   Dislocation of the articular processes

Currently, the most widespread, generally accepted classification of spinal injuries is the AO/ASIF classification developed by Magerl F. (1998), which is an international standard. According to this classification, three types of injuries are distinguished - A, B, C. (Fig. 5). Type - A - compression fractures (includes both stable and unstable fractures), Type - B - distraction (unstable) fractures, Type - C - complex torsional injuries (fracture-dislocations).

In AO classification, a two-column model is used and three categories of damage are distinguished.

A. vertebral compression

B. Damage to anterior and posterior structures due to stretching

C. Damage to anterior and posterior structures due to rotation

Each category is further divided into 9 subtypes using the classic 3-3-3 scheme.

AO-classification of injuries of the thoracolumbar junction
(according to Magerl 1994).

Vertebral body compression	
A1	Puncture fractures
A2	Splinter fractures
A3	Blast fractures
Damage to anterior and posterior structures due to stretching	
B1	Flexion-distraction predominantly ligamentous
B2	Flexion-distraction predominantly bony
B3	Hyperextension
Damage to anterior and posterior structures due to rotation	
C1	Type A with rotation
C2	Type B with rotation

<table><tr><td>C3</td><td>Damage due to shear rotation</td></tr></table>

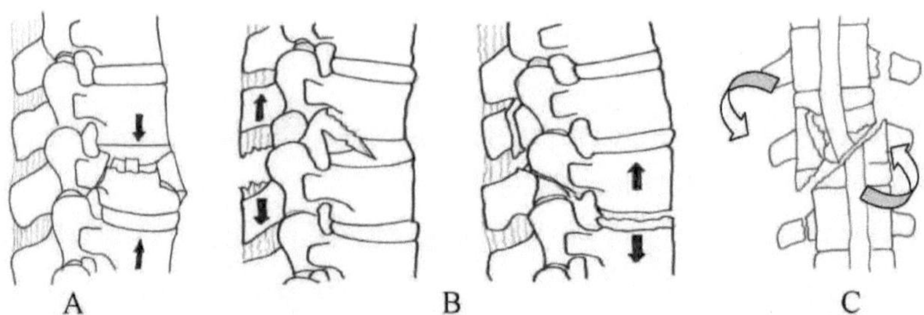

Figure 5. Three types of spinal injuries according to the AO/ASIF classification. A - compression fractures; B - distraction fractures; C - complex torsional injuries (fracture-dislocations).

Each of these types of injuries has its own varieties, which are categorized into groups. Thus, in group A, which according to the AO/ASIF classification belong to compression fractures, one can see both "typical" stable compression fractures and frontal and unstable fragility fractures (Fig. 6 a,b,c).

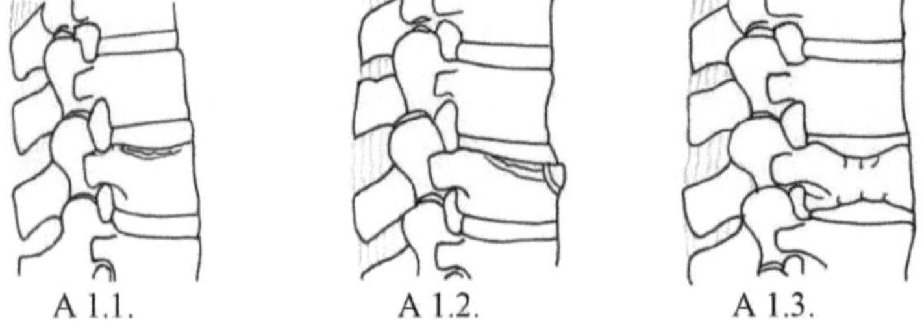

Figure 6a. A 1.1. Compression at the level of the closure plate. A 1.2. Wedge-shaped injury to the vertebral body. A 1.3. Double-concave (collapse) compression of the vertebral body.

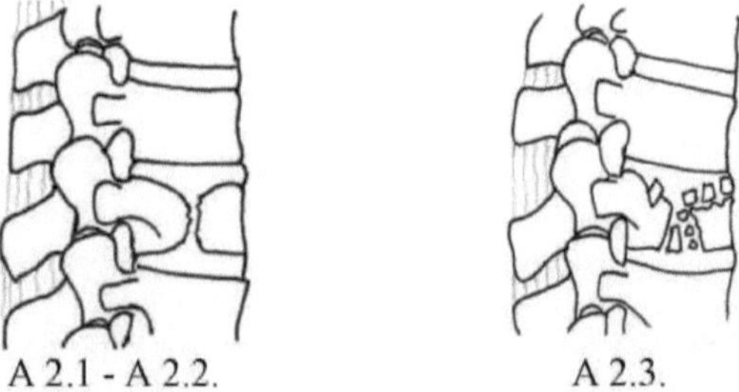

Fig. 6b. A 2.1 - A 2.2. - Fracture with splitting of the vertebral body in the sagittal or frontal plane. A 2.3. Vertebral body fracture with splitting of the vertebral body in the frontal and sagittal planes with fragmentation.

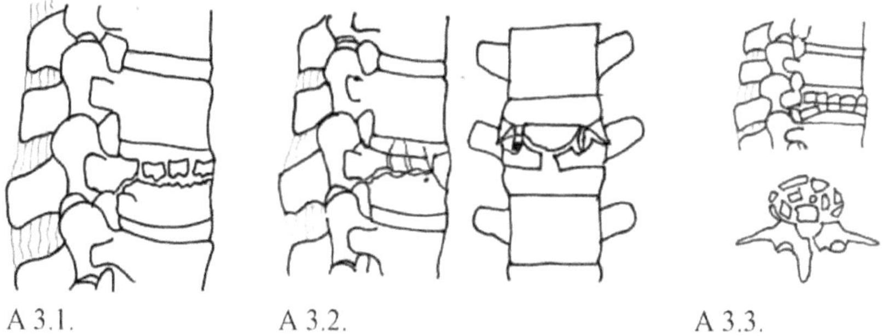

A 3.1.   A 3.2.   A 3.3.

Fig.6c. A3.1. Incomplete blast fracture. A3.2. Explosive fracture with splitting. A 3.3. Complete explosive fracture.

Type "B" includes unstable fractures and fracture-dislocations of predominantly flexion or extension mechanism as well as extension mechanism (Fig.7 a,b,c).

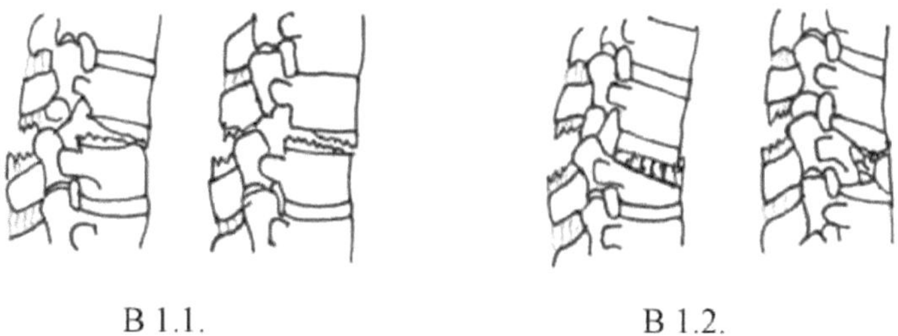

B 1.1.   B 1.2.

Figure 7a. B1.1 Posterior ligamentous injury in combination with transverse disc rupture. B1.2 Posterior ligamentous injury combined with type A vertebral body fracture.

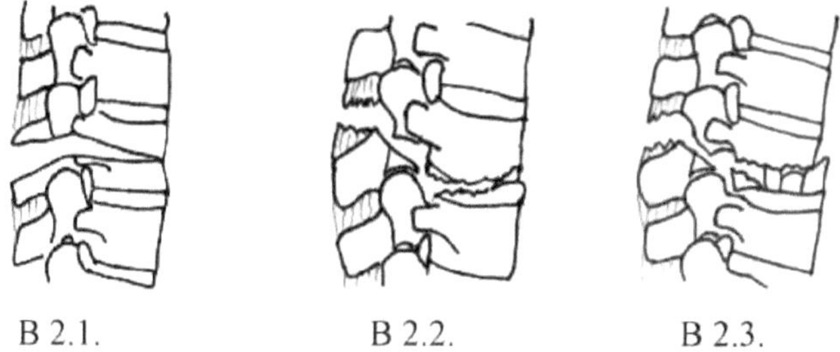

B 2.1.   B 2.2.   B 2.3.

Fig.7b. B2.1. Transverse fracture of both columns. B2.2 Damage to the posterior column (predominantly bony structures) with transverse disc fracture. B2.3 Damage to the posterior column (predominantly bony structures) in combination with a type A vertebral body fracture.

15

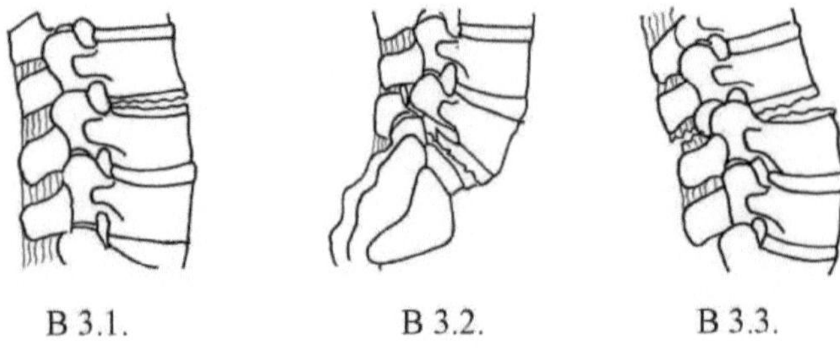

B 3.1.   B 3.2.   B 3.3.

Fig.7c. B3.1 Hyperextension subluxation. B3.2 Hyperextension spondylolysis. B3.3. Lesion with posterior displacement.

Type C includes the most severe injuries in terms of mechanism and heavy destruction of anatomical structures. In the pathomechanism of these injuries, rotational violence or shear violence plays an important and sometimes leading role (Fig. 8 a,b,c,d).

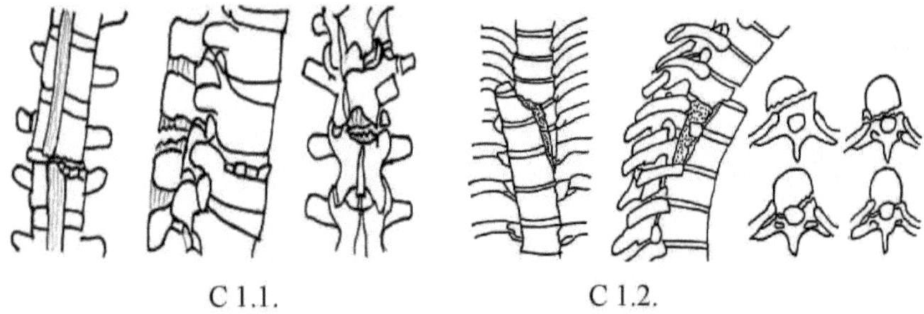

C 1.1.   C 1.2.

Fig.8a. C1.1 Rotational wedge fracture. C1.2. Vertebral body separation.

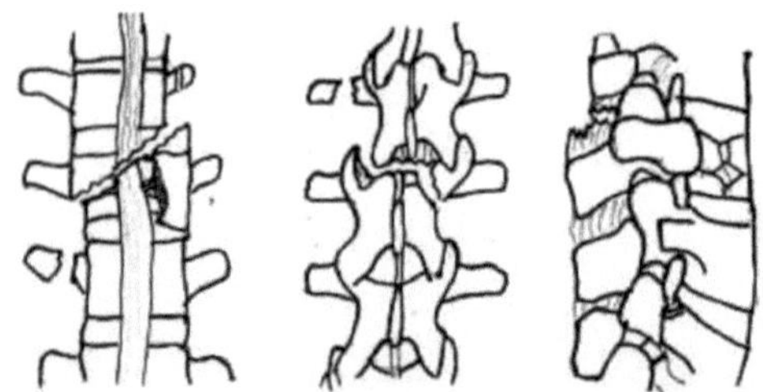

Fig.8b. C1.3. Complete explosive fracture of type A with rotation.

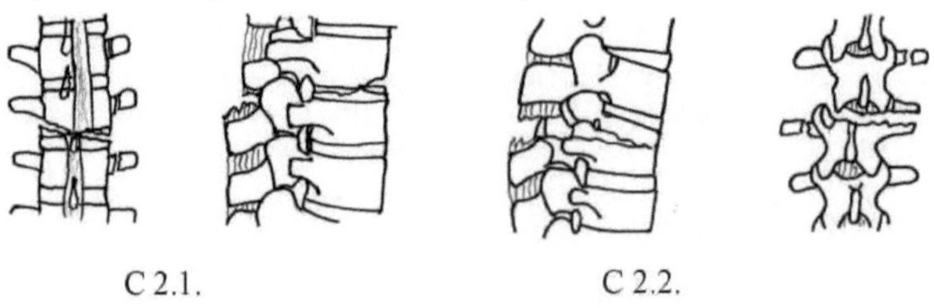

C 2.1.   C 2.2.

Fig.8c. C2.1. Type B injury with rotation - rotatory flexion subluxation. C2.2. Type B injury with rotation - transverse fracture of both columns with rotation.

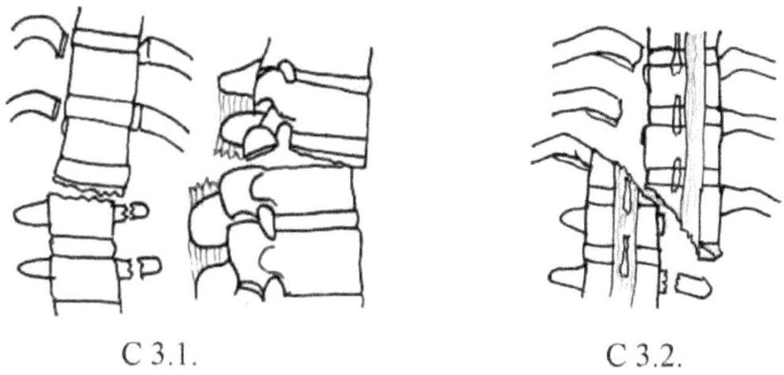

C 3.1.   C 3.2.

Fig.8g. C3.1 Rotational fracture - Holdsworth shearing fracture. C3.2 Rotational fracture - oblique spinal fracture.

Radiation assessment of spinal cord injury

Radiation evaluation of spinal cord injury includes conventional x-rays, computed tomography (CT) and magnetic resonance imaging (MRI). The purpose of radiation assessment is to: determine the localization and extent of the injury, identify signs of instability, classify the nature of the fracture, determine the extent of damage to the integrity of the spinal canal and elements of spinal cord compression, and determine the multiplicity of spinal injury.

Plain radiographs in two standardized projections (anteroposterior and lateral) of good quality should be performed in all patients with suspected spinal injury. The appropriate x-ray is performed based on the patient's complaints of spinal pain, localized soreness or deformity, and the presence of neurologic abnormalities.

In certain situations, it is not always possible to rotate the patient and, therefore, rotations of the X-ray tube on the machine should be used for lateral projection of the object.

There are three areas that require special skills in radiography and interpretation of radiographs: the upper cervical spine, the cervicothoracic spine, and the lumbosacral spine. To identify lesions in the area of the C1 vertebrae, radiographs in direct projection through an open mouth are required (you can use a tube used for dental radiography). The contours of the vertebrae in these areas on radiographs may not be clearly traced as a result of layering of surrounding bone formations: at the level of the first cervical vertebra, the bones of the skull are layered, at the cervical-thoracic level - the bones of the shoulder girdle, at the fifth lumbar vertebra - the bones of the pelvis. In the thoracolumbar region, the T12-L1 vertebral bodies are often indistinctly contoured due to layering of the liver shadow.

Computed tomography (CT) and magnetic resonance imaging (MRI) are the most informative in diagnosing violations of the integrity of the vertebral bone-disc and joint complex, as well as violations of the contours, shape and volume of the spinal canal. The information in these examination modalities, especially MRI, is so demonstrative and high resolution that it can be likened to layer-by-layer slices of a frozen preparation. Moreover, by performing the study in one plane, a three-dimensional image can be obtained as well as an image in three planes. CT is more informative for imaging bone tissue and its structure. MRI provides more information about the state of the surrounding soft tissues, discs and spinal canal contents on modes of different tissue density, and also provides an opportunity to obtain a contrast myelography image without contrast injection (Fig. 9). It should be noted that all these methods (radiography, CT and MRI) do not replace, but in some cases, complement each other.

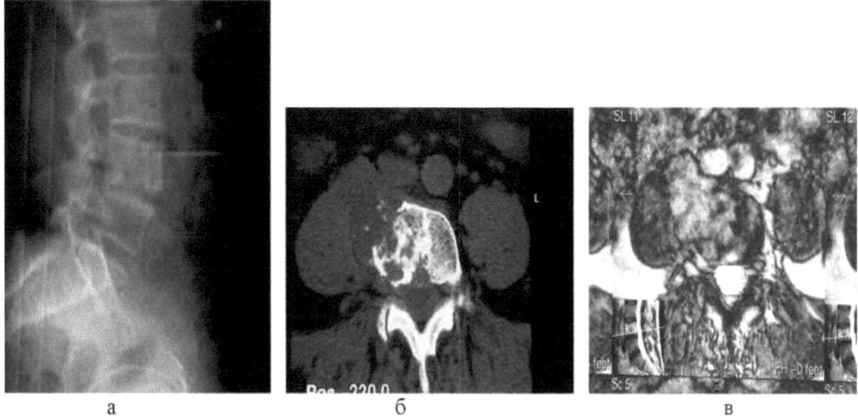

a   б   в

Figure 9. Image of the L4 vertebral tumor on radiograph (a), CT (b) and MRI (c).

The most important method of examination is radiologic. At the slightest suspicion of damage to the cervical spine, radiography in two mutually perpendicular projections: anteroposterior and lateral is mandatory. In some cases, the outlines of the lower cervical and first thoracic vertebrae can be identified only on CT.

For the upper cervical region (C1 - C2 vertebrae), the anteroposterior projection is performed through the open mouth in the supine position. Lateral projection is performed in the standard laying position. In this case, the radiograph shows the two upper vertebrae - C1 and C2 (atlantus and axis), articular facets and articular slits C1-C2. The lateral masses of the first vertebra can be seen, which lie laterally from the axis tooth in the form of two parallelograms. The symmetry of the above structures is disrupted when the injury occurs (Figs. 10, 11).

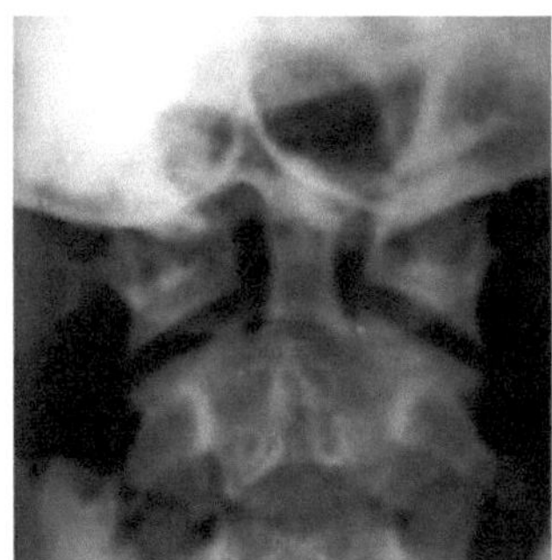

Figure 10. Radiograph of the C1-C2 vertebrae through an open mouth.

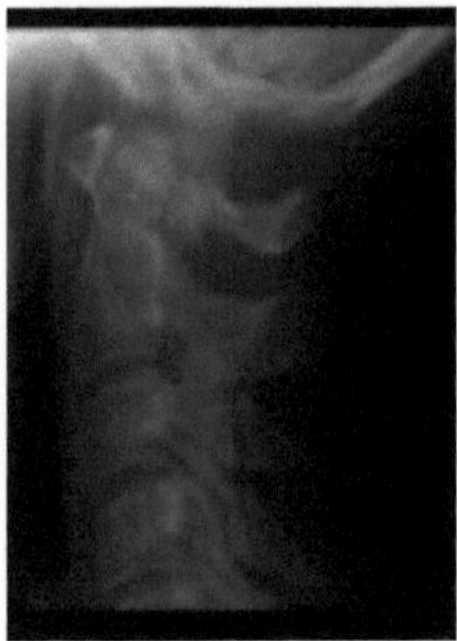

Fig.11. Anatomical formations on the lateral radiograph of the upper cervical spine: - occipital bone, - anterior and posterior arches of the atlantus, - C2 denticle, - C2 body, - C2 isthmus and sulcus

Suboccipital fractures

1. atlanto-occipital dislocation - the result of stretching and displacement of the ligamentous complex between the skull and the cervical spine, CT scan shows an increase in the distance between the basion and the dentate process of more than 12mm.

Dislocations of the head at the atlanto-occipital joint occur as a result of massive trauma and are accompanied by craniocerebral injuries. Patients are in a severe, often unconscious state, or die on the spot. Therefore, in clinical practice, these cases are rare and belong to the category of casuistry. Diagnosis is possible on lateral projection radiographs (Fig. 12).

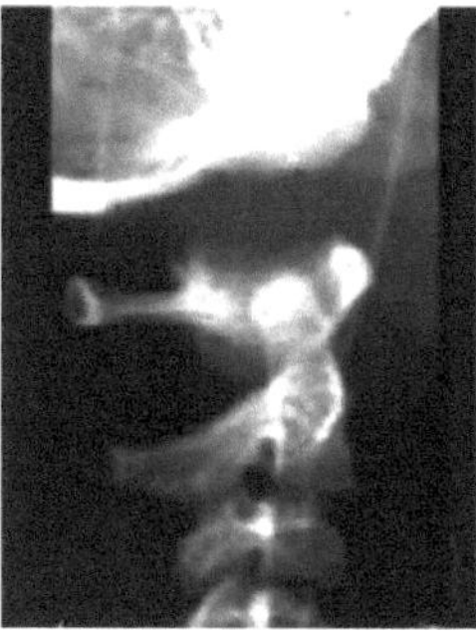

Fig.12. Dislocation at the atlanto-occipital joint: significant separation of the articular surfaces of the occipital bone and the atlantus can be seen.

This may also include fractures of the articular condyle of the occipital bone, detectable on CT (Figure 13).

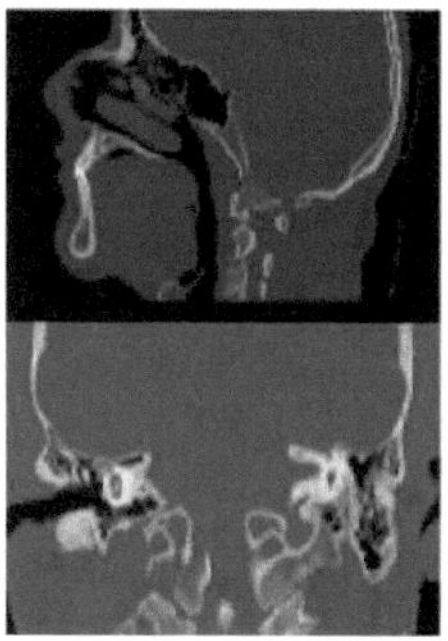

Figure 13. CT scan of the skull base and upper spine. A fracture of the articular condyle of the occipital bone is identified

C1 fractures are categorized into 5 subtypes based on the course of the fracture line.

Type I	Anterior arch fracture	Often combined with a fracture of the C2 dentition
Type II	Posterior arch fracture	The most common fracture
Type III	Jefferson's fracture	Unstable bilateral symmetrical

		fracture of the anterior and posterior arches, always with transverse ligament rupture
	Type I	No fragment displacement
	Type II	Anterior displacement and angled anterior arch displacement
	Type III	Optional front and
		cranial displacement of the posterior arch
Type IV	Lateral mass fracture	
Type V	Transverse process fracture	

Atlantus fractures, like other vertebrae, can be stable or unstable. They are categorized into 4 types based on the nature of the fracture. If the vertebral arch fractures in one place, the fracture will be stable. If fractured in two or more places, the fracture is unstable (Figure 3, Figure 15). Such a fracture of the first cervical vertebra is called a burst or cracking fracture (Jefferson fracture). In this case, the annulus atlantis bursts like a bagel and its lateral masses diverge laterally as a result of axial loading, as the head is inclined into the first cervical vertebra at the time of injury with force applied to the head along the axis of the trunk. The leading diagnostic value is radiography performed through an open mouth in a straight projection. The displacement of the lateral masses of the atlantus relative to the axis tooth and their overhanging over the axis body are noted. The exact diagnosis of the vertebral fracture itself and its nature are possible on CT scan.

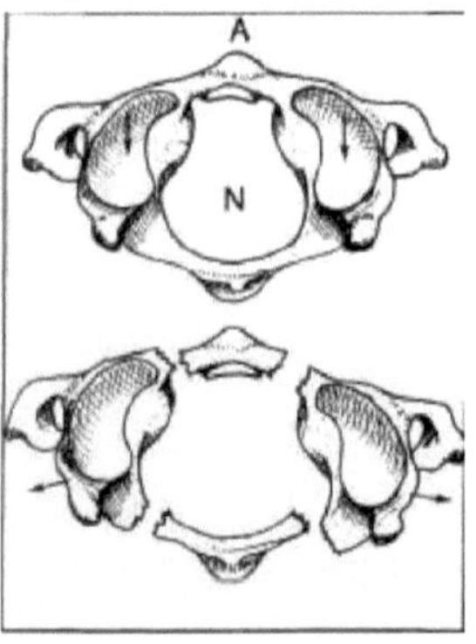

Figure 14. Fracture of the 1st cervical vertebra (Jefferson burst fracture).

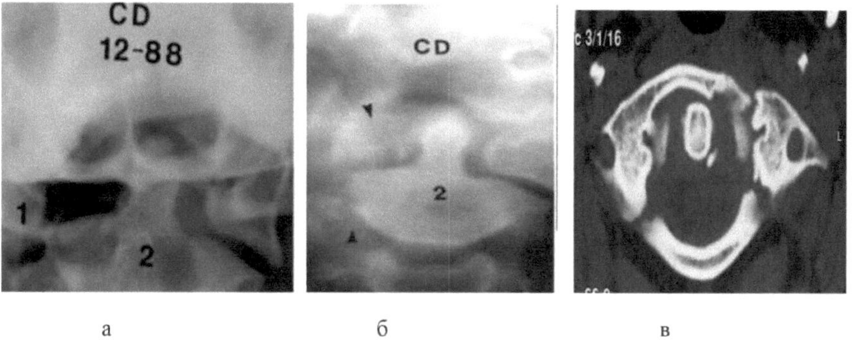

Fig. 15. Jefferson's fracture; a - open mouth radiograph: the right lateral mass (1) is displaced to the right; b - the same picture on CT scan - arrows indicate fractures of the atlantar arch and lateral masses of the vertebral body (2); c - CT scan - fracture of the anterior and posterior atlantar arch (Jefferson's fracture).

Type I-II fractures (schematically).

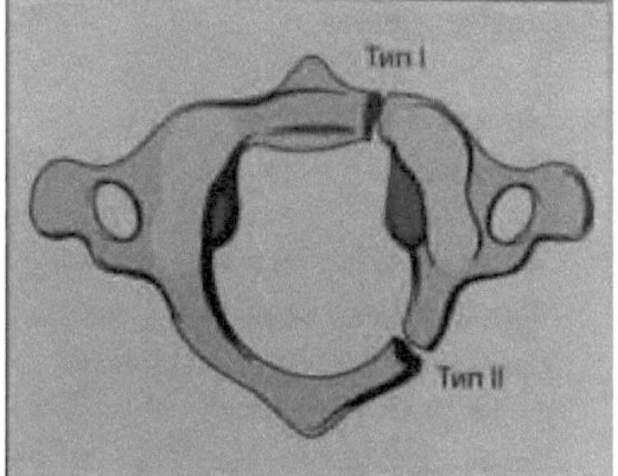

Jefferson fracture (type III).

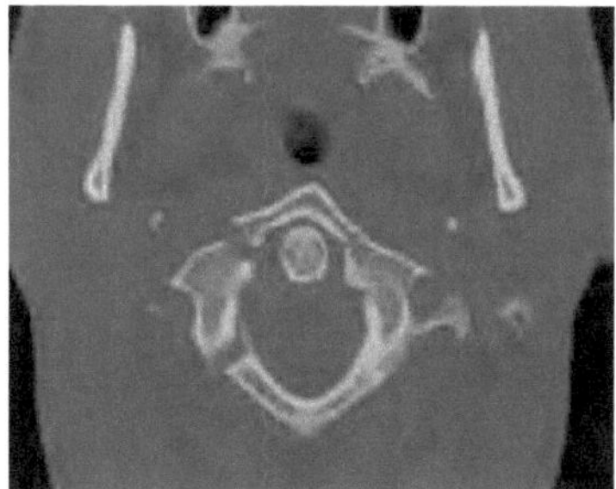

C1 fracture (type IV).

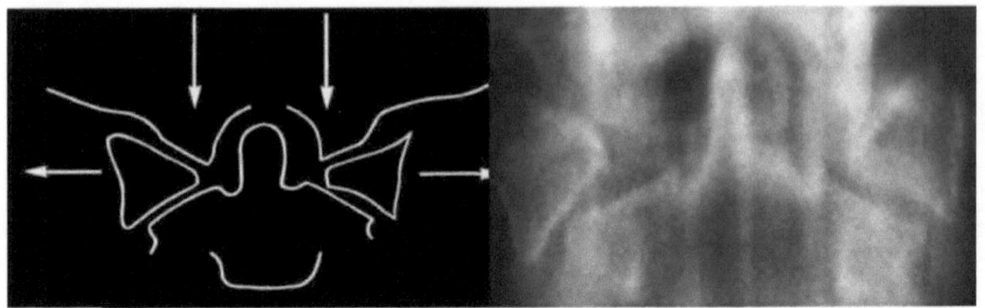

Lesions at the C1-C2 level should include subluxations of the atlas.

Rotational subluxations of the atlas

Atlantoaxial rotatory fixation is an irreparable posttraumatic subluxation. There are four degrees of its severity, of which II-IV are accompanied by rupture of the transverse ligament and enlargement of the atlanto-tooth space.

The radiographs show that the symmetry of the lateral masses of the atlas in relation to the dentition is broken. On the side of the subluxation, the distance from the tooth to the lateral mass of the atlas is greater than on the opposite side (Fig. 16). A lateral radiograph is not informative in these cases, but it is mandatory to exclude a fracture of the axis tooth base.

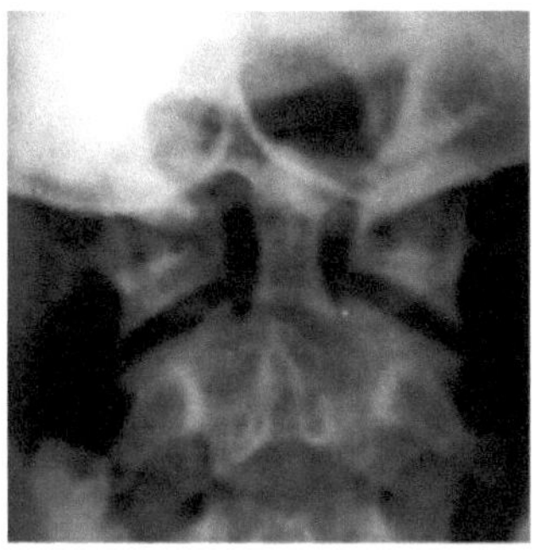

a

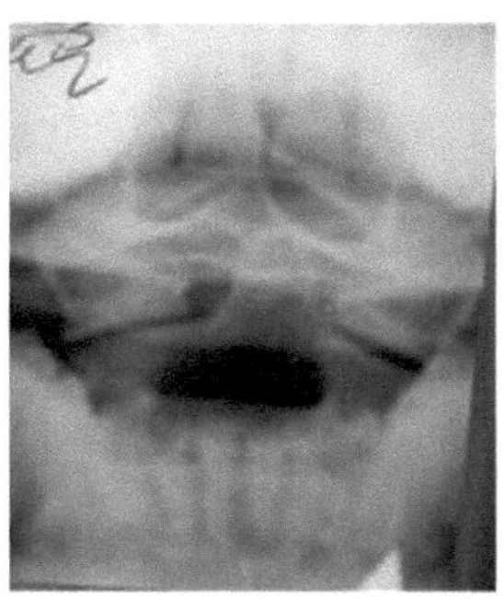

б

Figure 16. Rotational subluxation of the atlantus. Radiograph of C1 and C2 through an open mouth. a - normal vertebral element ratios: lateral masses of C1 are equally distant from the C2 tooth. b - rotational subluxation of C1 - lateral masses of C1 are not symmetrically located relative to the C2 tooth, the right articular gap is narrower than the left.

Transligamentary and peridental dislocation of the atlantus.

Transligamentary dislocation of the atlantus is caused by a rupture of the transverse ligament of the atlantus. In this case, the atlas and the head are displaced anteriorly, away from the dentition. Peridental dislocation is caused by the tooth slipping out from under the transverse ligament.

The main radiologic sign of transligamentary atlantoaxial dislocation is a widening of the articular gap of the anterior atlantoaxial joint (the joint between the posterior surface of the atlantoaxial arch and the anterior surface of the axis tooth - the Creuvillier joint). Normally, the gap does not exceed 2.5 mm. (Figure 17).

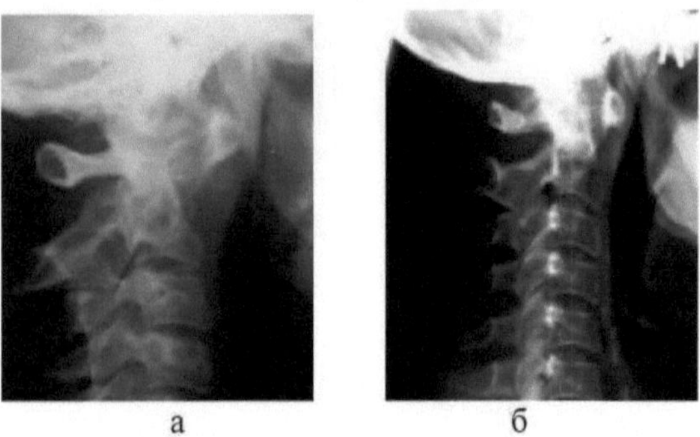

a   б

Fig.17 . Transligamentary dislocation of the atlas. The dentate process is intact. The first cervical vertebra with the head displaced anteriorly relative to C2. a - The articular crevilier joint gap is widened to one cm, b - The crevilier joint gap is greater than 2 mm.

C2 vertebral fractures

A fracture of the axis tooth in direct projection is characterized by a fracture line that may run through the apex of the tooth, as an arc-shaped serrated line from the apex of the tooth to the base, at the base of the tooth transversely, or entering the axis body (Fig. 18).

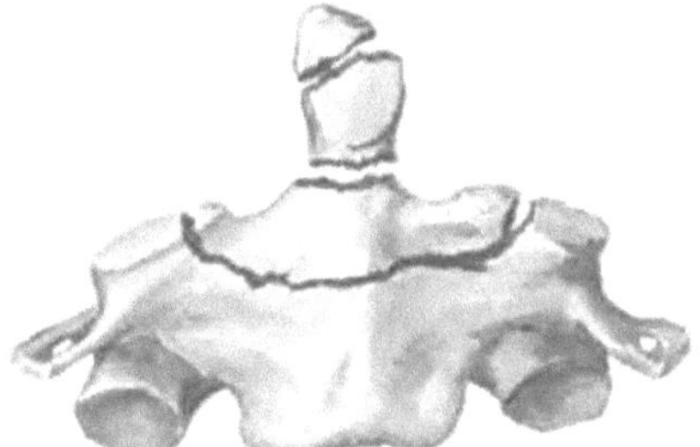

Fig.18. Axis tooth fracture: - fracture of the apex, - fracture at the base of the tooth, - fracture of the tooth with the upper part of the C2 vertebral body.

There are three degrees of misalignment of a broken tooth. The 1st degree of displacement is characterized by the tooth tilting a few degrees. The 2nd degree is characterized by displacement of the tooth in width by a few mm and inclination of the tooth to the front or back. In the third degree, the axis, together with the atlanto and head, is displaced anteriorly or posteriorly to the full width of the tooth (Fig. 19).

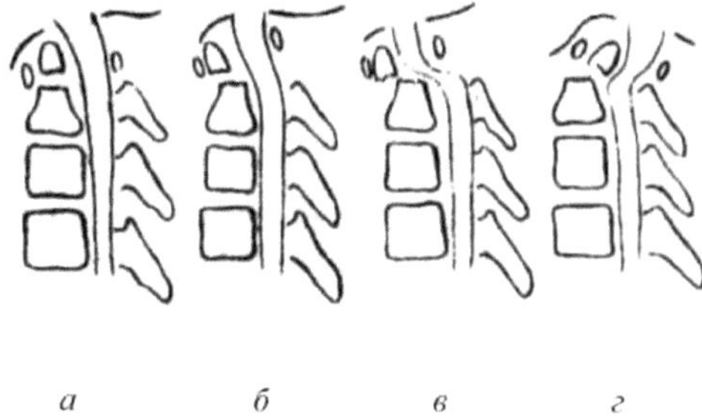

Fig.19. Axis tooth fracture (a - 1st degree; b - 2nd degree; c - 3rd degree; d - posterior displacement of the axis tooth).

A reliable sign of an axis tooth fracture on lateral projection radiographs is its anterior displacement along with the first vertebra. The anterior contour of the axis tooth forms a broken line with the anterior surface of the C2 vertebral body (Figs. 20, 21).

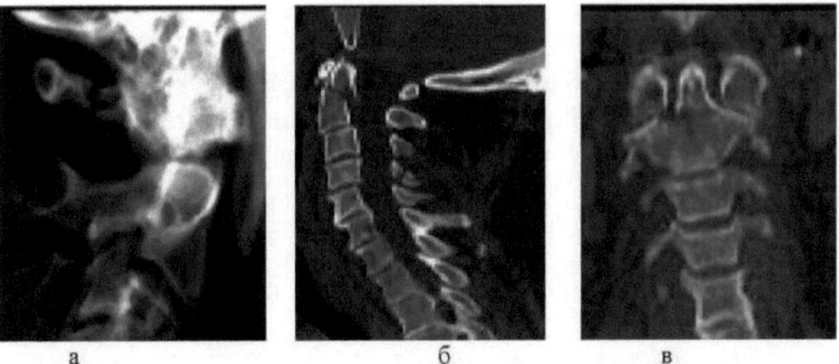

a   б   в

Fig.20. Fracture of the axis tooth. a - the radiograph shows a fracture of the posterior part of the atlantus arch and a fracture of the axis tooth without displacement. b - CT scan - fracture of the axis tooth at the base, posterior displacement of the tooth. c - CT direct projection - fracture of the axis tooth at the base.

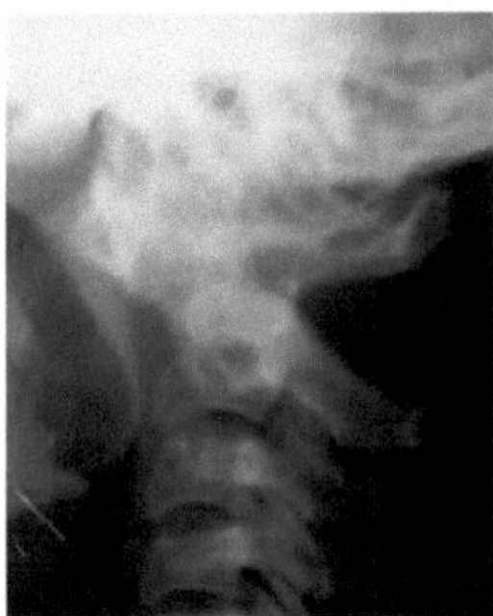

Figure 21. Axis tooth fracture with anterior displacement of ½ of its diameter. The anterior contour of the tooth and the C2 vertebral body form a broken line.

Distinguish between fractures of the dentition and so-called "hangman" fractures.

Fractures of the C2 vertebral dentition can be characterized fairly completely according to the Anderson and d*Alonzo classification and are usually due to hyperflexion injury, less frequently hyperextension injury (Fig.18).

Fractures of the C2 dentition (according to Anderson and d*Alonzo)

Type I	Fracture of the apex of the dentition (usually stable)
Type II	Fracture through the base of the dentition (unstable)
Type III	Fracture through the base of the dentition and the body of C2 (stable)

C2 "hangman" fractures (by Effendi)

Type I	Isolated axis arch fracture with displacement less than 3mm (stable)
Type II	Arch fracture with disc rupture and ventral displacement of the vertebral body C2 more than 4 mm and at an angle of more than 11 degrees (unstable)
Type III	Arch fracture with disc rupture and dislocation of the C2-C3 intervertebral

The next characteristic injury is fracture-dislocation of the C_2 , in which there is a fracture of the axis arch pedicle and displacement of its body together with the overlying spine and head to the front (traumatic spondylolisthesis). These injuries are figuratively called "hangman's fracture", "hangman's fracture". Displacement of the body may be minimal, 1 to 2 mm, or dislocation may occur almost to the width of the underlying vertebral body (Fig. 22)

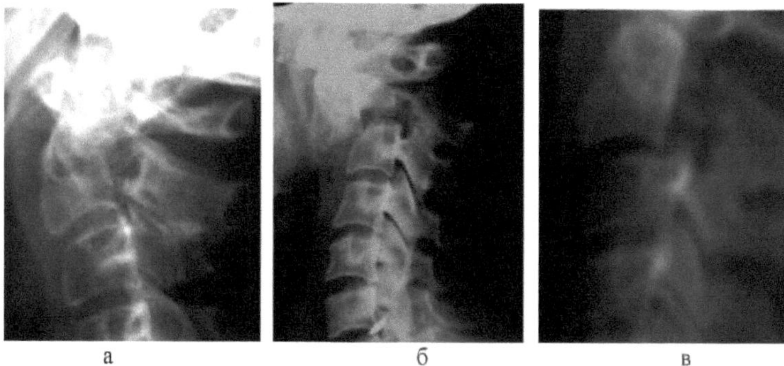

Fig.22. Fracture-dislocation of the C2 vertebra ("hangman's injury"): a - slight displacement of the C2 body; b - displacement of C2 over the entire width of the vertebral body, c - moderate (¼ part) displacement of the C2 body

Wedge compression fractures are less common in the cervical spine than in other parts of the spine. Vertebral body fragment fractures or a combination of an inferior vertebral body fracture and dislocation or subluxation of the superior vertebra are more common. According to Henle, there are 3 degrees of displacement of the articular surfaces: up to ¼ - I degree, up to half - II degree, up to 3/4 - III degree). There is also an IV degree of subluxation (dislocation) - superior dislocation. In an upper dislocation, the tips of the lower articular processes of the displaced vertebra are located on the tips of the upper articular processes of the vertebra below. When a vertebra is dislocated and the inferior articular processes of the displaced vertebra are positioned anterior to the superior articular processes of the underlying vertebra, it is commonly referred to as a fused dislocation (Figure 23).

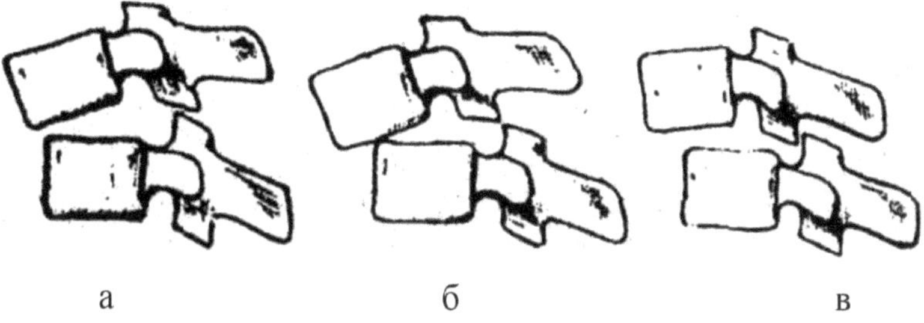

Fig.23. Vertebral dislocations: a - subluxation; b - superior dislocation; c - traction dislocation.

A distinction is made between tipping dislocations (with vertebral tilt) and sliding dislocations (without tilt, with displacement in the horizontal plane) (Figures 24, 25).

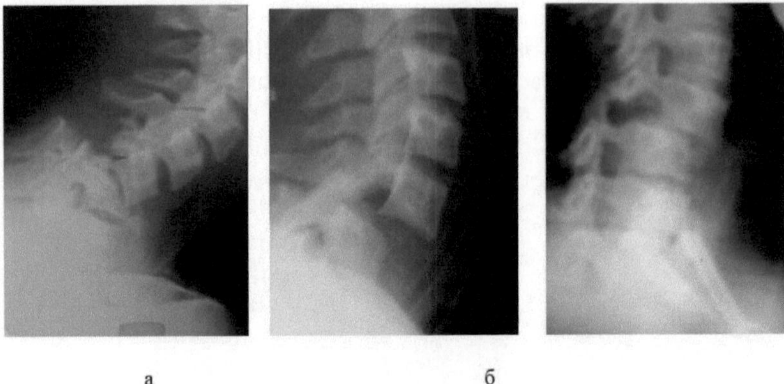

a   б

Fig.24. a - Tipping dislocation of the C5 vertebra. The vertebral body is tilted anteriorly relative to the underlying vertebra, and the posterior vertebral elements are destroyed. b - shearing dislocation. The displaced upper vertebra has blocked the spinal canal between its arch and the posterior-upper edge of the underlying vertebral body

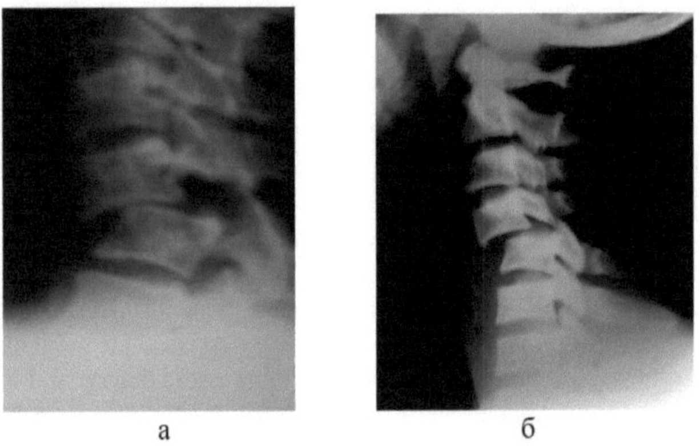

a   б

Fig.25. Varieties of vertebral dislocation. a - vertebral uppercuts, b - traction dislocation

Accurate diagnosis of spinal canal misalignment is possible with CT and MRI scans, which can determine the presence of a displaced intervertebral disc in the spinal canal, spinal cord involvement or surrounding fleshy tissues.

Tear-type fractures are defined as the detachment of a fragment of the anterolateral edge of a vertebra. They are caused by flexion trauma and are more often localized at the level of the C5-C7 vertebrae. These fractures are usually extremely unstable, accompanied by rupture of the anterior longitudinal ligament and result in dorsal displacement of the vertebral body. There is hemorrhage in the soft tissues in these fractures, which is visualized as an increase in their volume. These fractures are often accompanied by a mid-sagittal fracture of the vertebral body (Fig. 26).

30

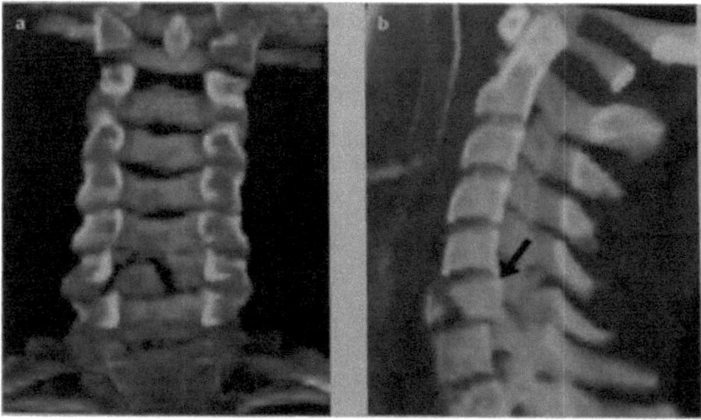

Figure 26. C6 tear-type fracture

Dugger fractures result from flexion trauma leading to a detachment fracture of the spinous process without ligamentous injury - these are stable fractures (Figure 27).

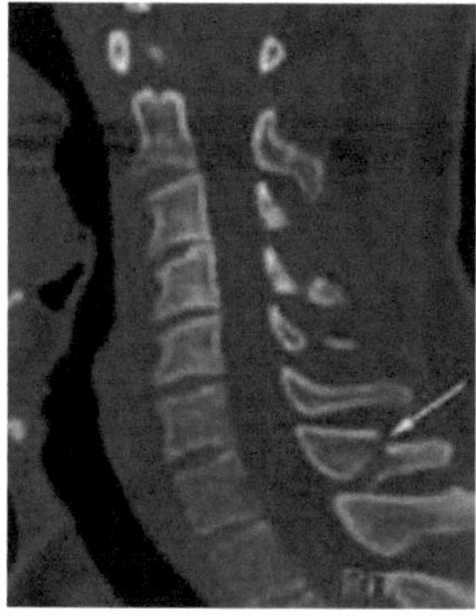

Figure 27. Digger fractures. Fracture of spinous process.

Explosive fractures of the cervical vertebrae occur after axial impact with rupture of the closure plates and penetration of the vertebral body by intervertebral disc fragments, the presence of a sagittal fracture line and multiple fragments. Their stability depends on the damage to the posterior surface of the vertebra, and displacement of fragments into the spinal canal is often determined.

Articular fractures are less common and are potentially unstable and require fixation. Cervical intervertebral joint dislocations: superior and traction are the result of extreme cervical flexion of the head and neck. These dislocations are usually unstable, often bilateral with ligamentous damage, and there is an anterior displacement of the cranial vertebra. Sagittal reformatting of the image is necessary to determine the presence of a traction dislocation and to assess the degree of narrowing of the intervertebral foramen. As a rule, images in the axial and sagittal planes complement each other and should be studied in an integrated manner.

Details of the nature and features of lesions in the cervical spine, as well as in other regions, are most accurately reflected on CT and MRI (Figures 28, 29).

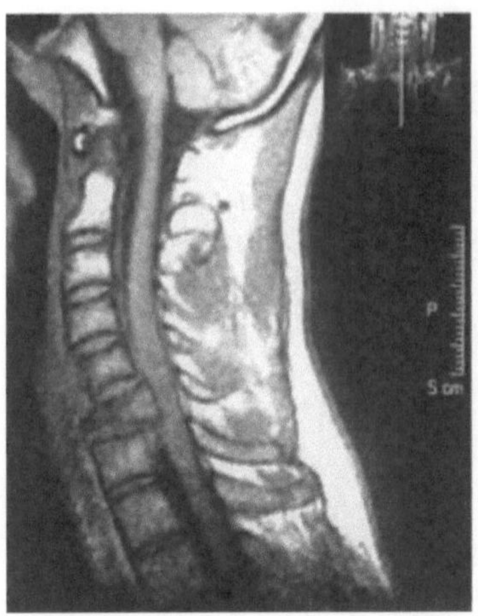

Figure 28: MRI image, blast fracture of the C6 vertebra.

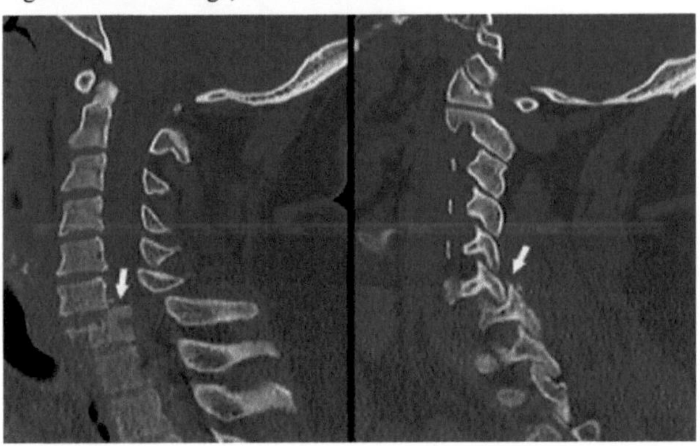

Figure 29: CT scan of the cervical spine: reveals a fracture with dislocation of the **C7** vertebra, facet joint fusion.

Injuries to the thoracic and lumbar spine.

The thoracic spine is the least susceptible to trauma due to the stability provided by the thoracic cage and occurs in severe trauma. The most common type of injury is flexion injury, given the anatomical features of the structure (physiologic kyphosis), which is accompanied by fracture-dislocations. The area of the thoracolumbar transition is more vulnerable to fractures. The main mechanisms of fractures in this zone are hyperflexion and compression, so compression fractures are the most common.

In trauma with displacement of fragments into the spinal canal, the degree of spinal canal stenosis should be assessed (Fig. 30).

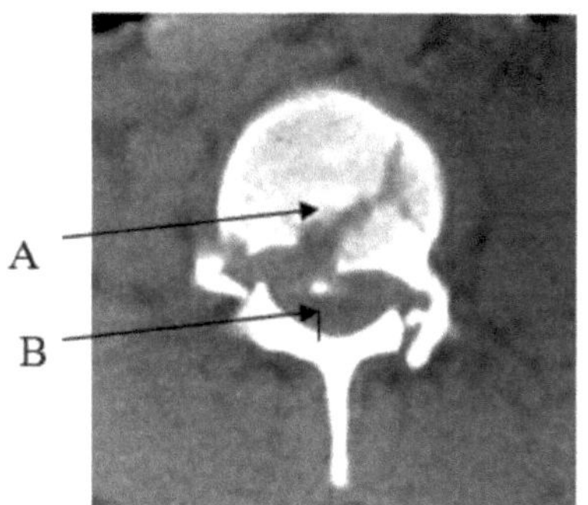
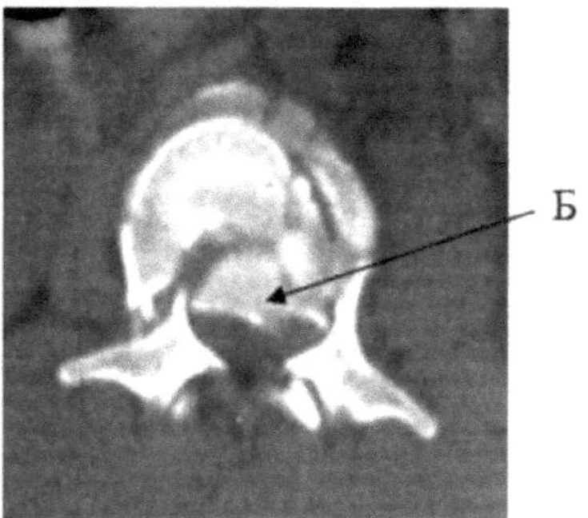

Figure 30. Explosive fracture of the vertebral body. Extrusion of fragments into the spinal canal. A - vertebral body, B - displaced fragment, C - vertebral arch.

The diagnosis of spinal canal stenosis is established by spondylometry on routine radiographs, computed tomograms (CT), magnetic resonance imaging (MRI) prints of the spine, and myelograms (MG). Of primary importance is the magnitude of the anteroposterior sagittal diameter of the spinal canal or dural sac. *A decrease in the distance from the posterior surface of the vertebral body to the nearest opposing point on the arch at the base of the spinous process of up to 12 mm in any spine segment is considered as spinal canal stenosis.* The radicular canal is considered narrowed if its minimum diameter at any level is equal to or less than 3 mm or if the radicular pocket is not contrasted at MG.

The spinal canal at different levels has a different cross-sectional area: on average 2.5 cm^2 , and the largest at the level of the fifth lumbar vertebra is 3.2 cm^2 .

The presence of contusions, hematomas, and spinal cord tears can only be reliably determined after an MRI.

In the radiologic diagnosis of spinal injuries, especially in the thoracic and lumbar spine, both on direct and profile radiographs, special attention should be paid to certain features that, by direct or indirect evidence, may indicate the nature of the fracture, the extent of the injury, and the appropriateness of the classification.

Widening of the interfemoral (intersternal) distance.

It is defined by the size of the straight line between the contours of the inner edge of the vertebral arches compared to this size of two adjacent vertebrae. An increase in this dimension indicates a vertebral body splinter fracture, which is a type A3/4 fracture (Figure 31).

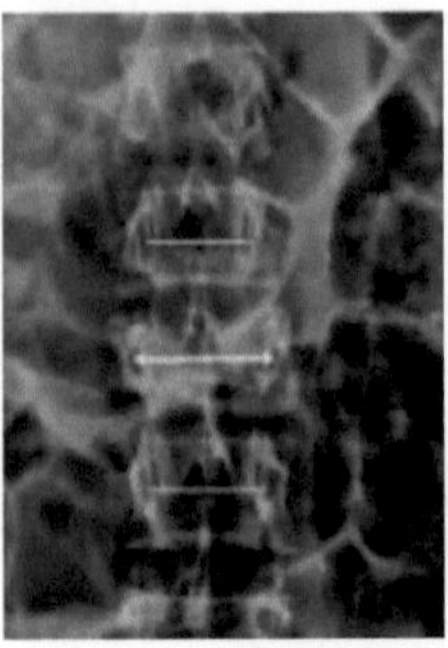

Figure 31: Increased interfemoral (interfemoral) distance indicates a splinter fracture - type A3/4

Lateral displacement of the vertebral body or altered spinous process relationships indicate vertebral displacement (subluxation or dislocation). This injury is classified as a type C injury. (Figure 32).

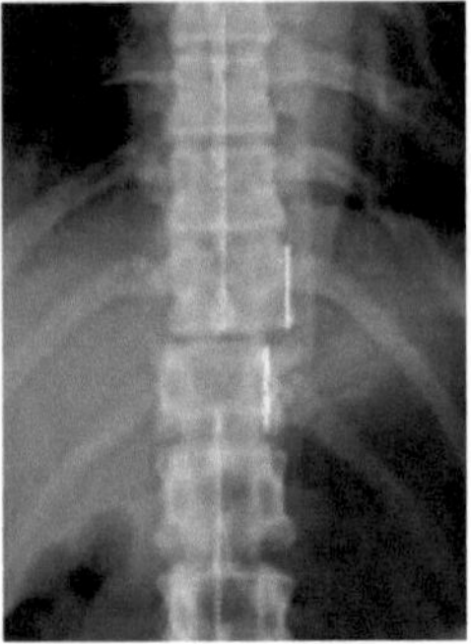

Figure 32: Lateral displacement of the vertebral body. The spinous process line is preserved. Type C injury.

An increase in the distance between the spinous *processes* (compared to adjacent levels) in the absence of lateral displacement indicates a distraction injury to the posterior vertebral elements - a Type B (B1 or B2) injury (Figure 33).

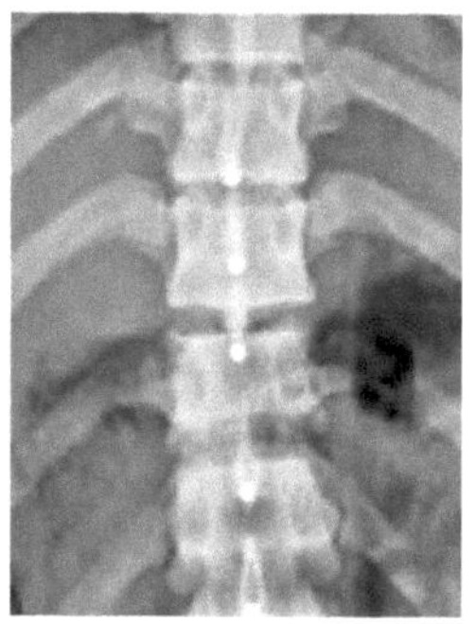

Figure 33: Increased distance between spinous processes (compared to adjacent levels) indicates distraction injury to the posterior vertebral elements. Type B injury (B1 or B2).

In some cases, a *horizontal slit (fracture line) in the vertebral body at the level of the pedicles* can be seen on high-quality direct projection radiographs. This is a sign of a distraction instability type B injury (Fig. 34).

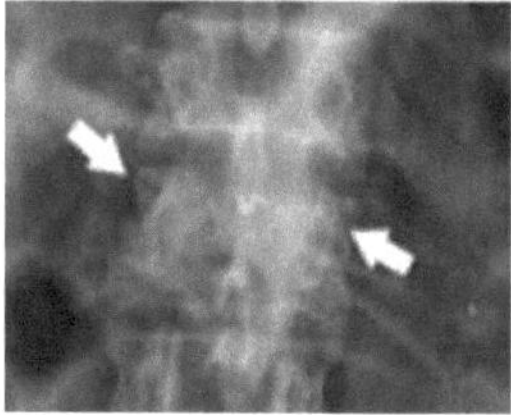

Figure 34: Horizontal slit (fracture line) in the body at the level of the pedicles. Fracture type B1.

While the interpretation of anteroposterior projection X-rays in spinal fractures is mostly focused on indirect signs of vertebral damage, profile radiographs clearly show signs of damage, which, together with fracture data on direct radiographs, allow for a more accurate, definite diagnosis.

Fractures with loss of anterior vertebral body height (the height of the anterior contour of the vertebral body measured along the anterior border of the spine from the inferior to the superior endplate and compared to the height of the adjacent normal vertebra) with preserved posterior vertebral body height are classified as type A injuries (Figure 35).

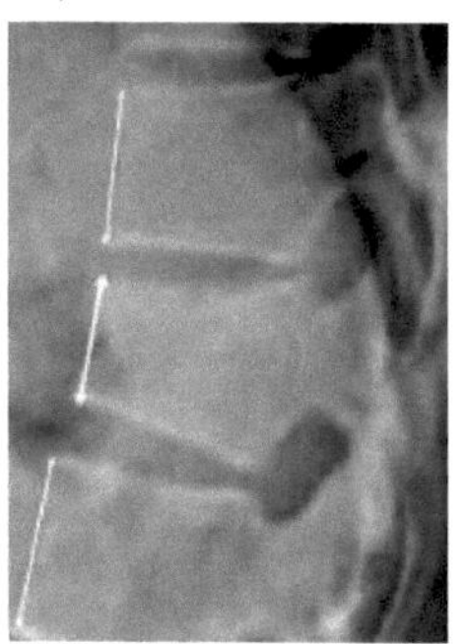

Figure 35. Loss of anterior vertebral body height. Measured along the anterior border of the vertebral body from inferior to superior endplate and compared to the height of the adjacent normal vertebra.

Vertebral body compression fractures are commonly categorized into three degrees depending on the degree of anterior vertebral body height reduction:

I st. - decrease in the anterior height of the vertebral body by 1/4;

II st. - Reduction of the anterior aspect of the vertebral body from 1/3 to 1/2 of the height;

III st.- decrease in the height of the anterior body more than ½.

Compression of the vertebral body II-IIICT. IS usually accompanied by kyphotic deformity, which may reach 30-40 or more degrees. The angle of deformation is determined by the intersection of two lines drawn along the posterior surface of the superior and inferior vertebrae. In this case, the inter-osteum is widened or the fracture line runs along the spinous process. In other words, there is trauma to the posterior support complex, which, together with the interest of the anterior and medial support, characterizes the fracture as unstable. Most of these fractures are type A (Figure 36).

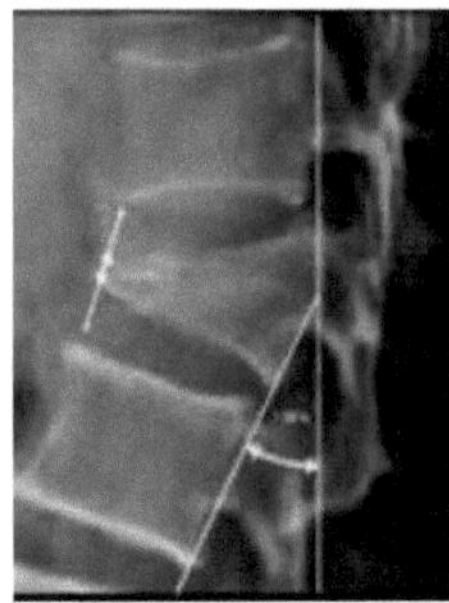

Figure 36: Vertebral body compression fracture Shst. Vertebral body compression >50%. Kyphosis >30 degrees.

The *degree of wedging of the vertebral body and the degree of loss of vertebral body height* can be determined using the formula for wedging index and vertebral body height loss index: **1cl** = hn : Hz, **1nv** = [^n:Hn)+ (bz:Hz)]:2, where: **1cl.** - is the index of vertebral body wedge shape, hn is the height of the anterior contour of the broken vertebra, Nz is the height of the posterior contour of the broken vertebra when its height is equal to the intact vertebra, **Ine** is the index of vertebral body height loss, Hn is the height of the anterior contour of the intact vertebra, hz is the height of the posterior contour of the broken vertebra (Fig. 37).

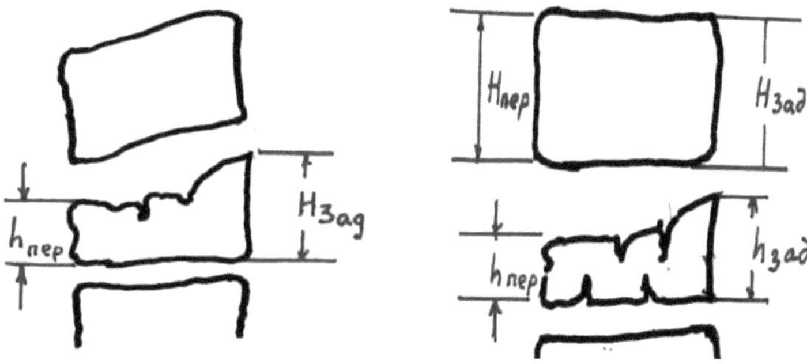

Figure 37: Schematic of the vertebral body wedge index (1cl) and vertebral body height loss index (1pv) (explained in the text).

Loss of height of the posterior contour of the vertebral body or disruption of the integrity of the posterior closure plate (the height of the posterior contour of the vertebral body is measured along the posterior portions of the vertebral border from superior to inferior end plate and compared to the adjacent normal vertebra) indicates marked compression of the vertebral body, involvement of the posterior wall of the vertebral body with possible extrusion of the fragment into the spinal canal - Type A3/A4. (Figure 38). In such cases, a CT scan is indicated to clarify the degree of bone trauma.

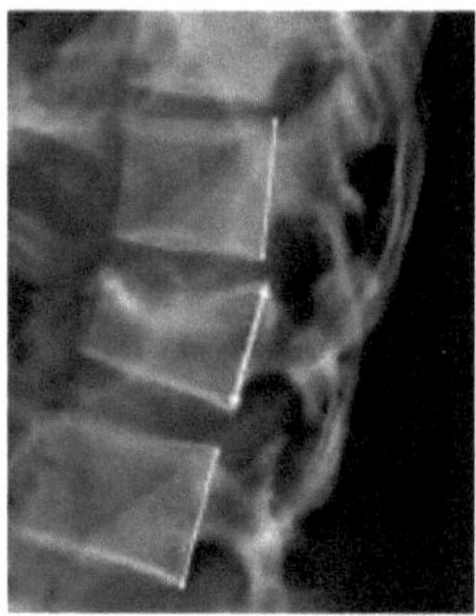

Figure 38: Loss of height of the posterior contour of the vertebral body indicates involvement of the posterior wall of the vertebral body with possible extrusion of the fragment into the spinal canal - Type A3/A4.

Loss of alignment (misalignment) of the vertebral bodies is interpreted as a subluxation. In these situations, subluxation or dislocation (fracture-dislocation) of the facet joints may be suspected. The lesions are classified as Type C (Figure 39).

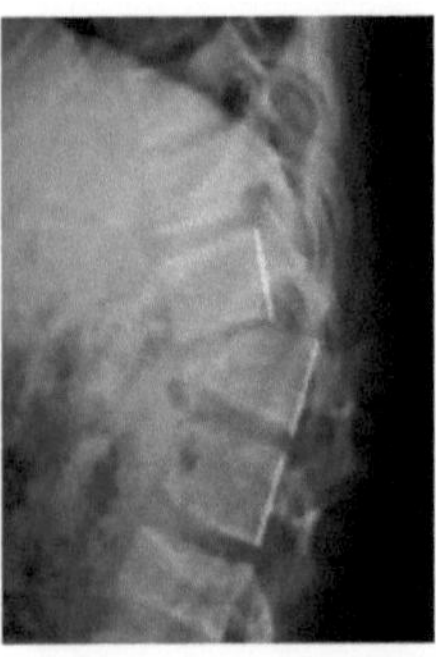

Figure 39: Dislocation (fracture-dislocation) of the superior vertebral body. Type C injury.

Type B distraction injuries present a peculiar picture. Kyphotic deformity with moderate wedge compression of the vertebral body may be accompanied by pronounced changes in the posterior osteo-ligamentous complex. This is a disconnection of the facet joints with an increase in the intercostal distance. This combination of injuries indicates damage to both anterior support structures and posterior support and is indicative of an unstable Type B2 fracture (Figure 40).

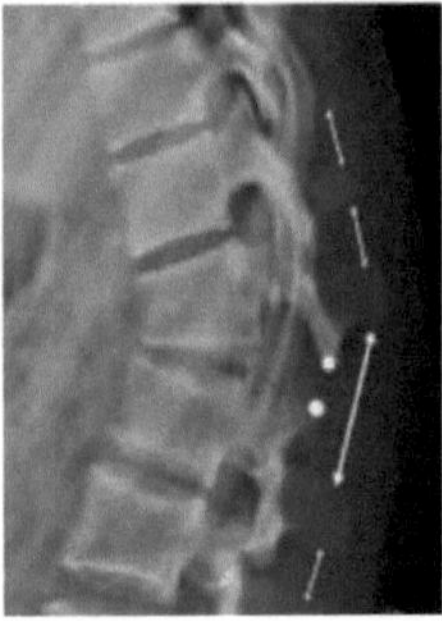

Figure 40. Type B2 fracture. Combination of wedge-shaped deformity of the vertebral body with facet joint separation and increased intercostal distance

At first glance, superficial injuries should be of concern in terms of severity of injury. *An isolated spinous process fracture indicates a stable type A-0 fracture.* However, *in the presence of an anterior A1 fracture, the presence of a horizontal spinous process fracture would indicate a type B1.2 injury.* Any such suspicion should warrant further CT examination (Figure 41).

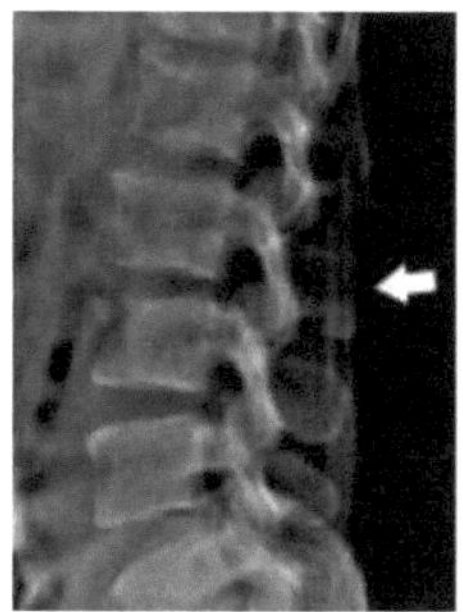

Figure 41: Type A1 fracture anteriorly, the presence of a spinous process fracture indicates a type B1.2 injury.

Computed and magnetic resonance tomography in the diagnosis of traumatic spinal cord injuries

CT and MRI scans provide important information about the extent and nature of damage in patients with spinal cord injury.

In modern trauma centers, CT is accepted as a screening method. Multidetector computed tomography (MDCT), depending on the nature of the injury, includes examination of the brain and bones of the skull, chest and abdominal organs, small pelvis with mandatory study of bone and traumatic changes. On modern devices from the first scan it is possible to obtain thin slices (less than one millimeter) necessary for the construction of optimal reconstructions with subsequent detailed analysis of traumatic skeletal lesions.

In spinal trauma, fractures come to the forefront, so it is not enough to analyze the whole body in detail, especially if thick slices were used. If a spinal fracture is suspected, a targeted thin-slice examination is mandatory.

In spiral CT, clinical symptoms (pain, neurologic prolapse), as well as the presence of paravertebral and retroperitoneal hematomas are the reason for detailed study of the adjacent vertebrae with thin slices in the bone window, with construction of multiplanar and volumetric reconstructions.

The questions that MDCT should answer are the stability of the fracture and the degree of compression of the spinal cord and spinal nerves. In spinal cord injury, the cervical and thoracolumbar spine are most commonly affected. Flexion and extensional injuries occur predominantly in the cervical spine, while compression injuries occur in the thoracic and lumbar spine. Fractures of the C1 and C2 vertebrae represent a separate category.

Vertebral fractures are often accompanied by edema of paravertebral soft tissues, and MPR reconstructions are used to assess the degree of edema.

In postoperative patients, CT scans are used to assess the spinal axis, the relationship between the vertebral bodies, and the degree of spinal canal stenosis. CT scanning provides necessary information after internal fixation and bone grafting surgeries to assess the position of implants, transpedicular screws, possible disruption of their position or integrity, "subsidence" of vertebral bodies, the presence of inflammatory changes and the degree of consolidation.

In trauma patients, it is usually preferable to scan one or another part of the spine as a whole to ensure high-quality MPR and 3D reconstructions. Collimation for the cervical spine is 0.5-2mm, for the thoracic spine 0.75-2mm, and for the lumbar spine 1-2.5mm. MDCT allows scanning of the entire spinal column in thin slices, which is of particular importance in patients with polytrauma. Scanning the entire spine as a whole is easier and allows for periformity in any plane exactly parallel to the plane of the injured vertebra or intervertebral disc, even in the presence of scoliosis. Such a scan certainly results in a certain increase in radiation exposure.

When creating image reconstructions, a small field of view is used to ensure optimal spatial resolution. In trauma patients, a high-resolution reconstruction algorithm (bone mode) is used, while a standard reconstruction algorithm should also be used to visualize adjacent soft tissues. When studying intervertebral disc injuries, a smoothing reconstruction algorithm is used to ensure a lower noise level in the images. A high-resolution algorithm is reasonable to use to evaluate the spinal canal and intervertebral foramen while performing reformatting in the sagittal, parasagittal, and frontal planes. For the cervical spine it is necessary to reformat with a slice thickness of no more than 1.5 mm, for the thoracic and lumbar spine it is acceptable to reformat with a slice thickness of 2-3 mm, which allows to reduce noise in the images.

In the cervical region, the image quality can be significantly reduced due to noise from the shoulder girdle, so to improve the quality of the images obtained, adaptive filtering is used; in modern CT scanners, the program automatically changes the exposure dose depending on the thickness of the object under study in different planes. As an alternative, MRI can be used in the study of the cervicothoracic junction, devoid of the above-mentioned disadvantages, but its use also has its limitations.

When multidetector spiral computed tomography is planned, conventional radiologic examination is currently rejected because it leads to increased radiation exposure, temporarily prolongs the examination, and, most importantly, does not provide additional information (and can sometimes cause misinterpretation of existing lesions). In addition, MDCT is much more sensitive in showing fractures and displacements than radiography and makes it possible to avoid underestimating the severity of injuries, to classify injuries into stable and unstable and to choose an adequate treatment. In patients with suspected instability or stenosis of the spinal canal, MDCT is necessary for planning surgical intervention, but if spinal cord injury is suspected, the patient's examination should be complemented by magnetic resonance imaging (MRI), which is also indicated for evaluation of the disco-ligamentous complex. MRI is also the best diagnostic modality for the cervical spine because it eliminates artifacts from the upper shoulder girdle.

Individual vertebral elements may not be visible on radiographs, and in transitional regions such as craniocervical, cervicothoracic, thoracic, thoracolumbar, and lumbosacral, images may be indistinct due to the layering of shadows of surrounding tissue structures. Numerous studies show that fractures are not visible on conventional radiographs in more than 20% of patients. Therefore, CT scans are routinely part of the examination plan in many centers. CT scans are especially necessary for the evaluation of a fracture according to the AO classification (AOSpine classification). Advantages of CT: most accurate representation of bony damage, sensitivity and specificity >95%, multispiral CT of the chest, abdomen and pelvis is available for visceral injury.

In addition to identifying the severity and nature of the vertebral injury, CT scans are extremely important in determining the relationship disruption in the spinal canal.

CT images clearly visualize a multifocal injury to the vertebral body. In addition to the degree of vertebral body fracture, displacement of the fragments, including into the spinal canal, can be determined. From these data, the degree of spinal canal involvement can be determined and accurately classified according to the AOSpine classification (Figure 42).

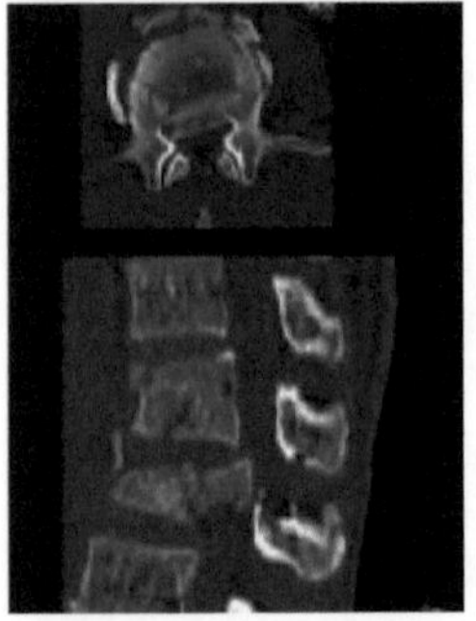

Figure 42: CT images show a multifocal vertebral body injury with displacement of the fragments into the spinal canal.

Axial CT scans provide additional information about the nature and size of fragments displaced into the spinal canal and the degree of spinal stenosis.

The normal sagittal dimension is determined by the average of the sagittal diameter of the spinal canal of the superior and inferior vertebrae. The percentage expression of the degree of narrowing of the spinal canal from baseline is determined by the formula: $A = (1 - x/y) \times 100$, where A is the percentage of narrowing, x is the smallest dimension of the spinal canal at the level of the lesion, and y is the average value of the mean sagittal dimension in a given patient (Fig. 43). T. Hashimoto et al. showed that spinal canal stenosis greater than 35% can lead to spinal cord injury or involvement, and many authors now use this concept to determine the indications or contraindications for surgical treatment.

Additional information about the degree of spinal stenosis is provided by determining the volume (area) of spinal stenosis. P.A. Rasmussen defined the critical area of the spinal canal at the level of L1 as 1 square centimeter (stenosis $\approx$ 67%). All patients with such an area of the spinal canal had paraplegia.

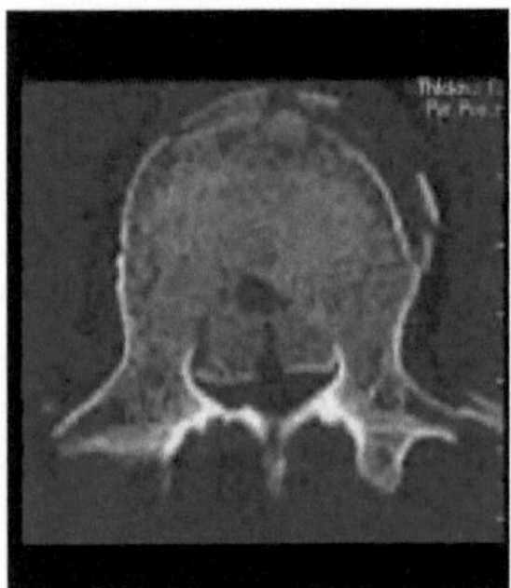

Fig.43. CT scan - axial projection. Protrusion of two bone fragments into the spinal canal.

Of particular importance is not only the degree of spinal stenosis, but also the specific characteristics of the fragments displaced into the spinal canal. In severe spinal trauma, at the moment of force application, the fragments not only rush into the spinal canal, but also rotate along their axis. This feature is of particular importance, as it indicates that it is impossible to correct the position by ligamentotaxis and requires only open decompression of the spinal canal (Fig. 44).

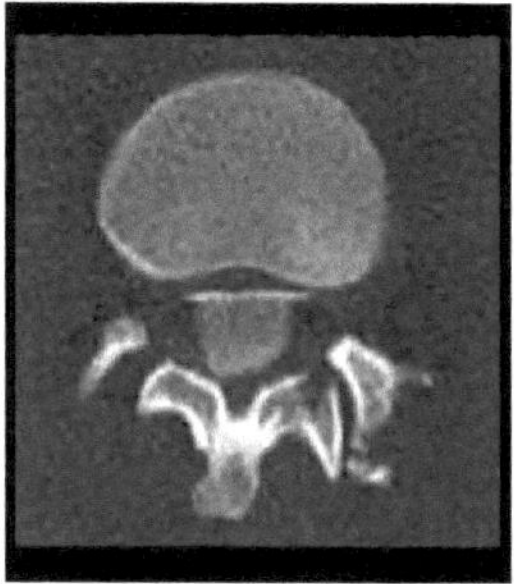

Figure 44. CT scan - axial projection. Reverse position (reversal) of the cortical plate (the displaced fragment is rotated 180 degrees so that its cortical surface opposes the surface of the main vertebral body).

The fragments displaced into the spinal canal may not be represented by one or two large fragments, but may be multifragmentary, indicating possible damage to the dura mater and impingement of nerve roots (Fig. 45).

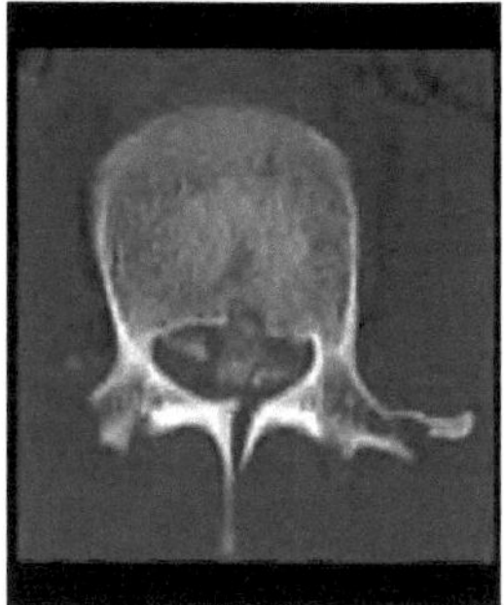

Figure 45. Multifragmentary pattern of fragments displaced into the spinal canal.

The CT scan may show a transpedicular fracture. Despite the seemingly small area of injury, this factor on the one hand indicates the unstable nature of the injury and on the other hand surgeons should avoid inserting screws into this area during transpedicular fixation (Fig. 46).

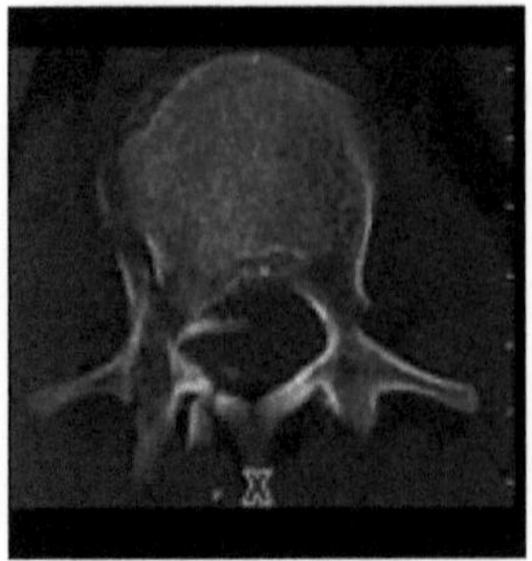

Figure 46. CT SCAN. Axial projection. Bilateral transpedicular fracture, arch fracture, displacement of the fragment into the spinal canal.

MRI study

MRI provides a great deal of information about the extent of soft tissue damage that occurred during spinal trauma. However, the need to stay in a forced position for a long time, the severity of the patient's condition with unstable hemodynamics, cases with polytrauma exclude the possibility of using MRI in all cases of spinal trauma in the acute period. In neurologic involvement, MRI accurately shows the degree of spinal cord compression, edema, hemorrhage, and the presence of transverse spinal cord injury. MRI also reveals posterior ligamentous complex injuries, disco-ligamentous complex injuries. MRI helps to detect multilevel injuries of non-contiguous segments. It is known that the degree of vertebral body compression and traumatic kyphosis may increase in the absence of proper fixation and sparing. The risk of progression remains during the first few months due to the initial regeneration processes characterized by bone repair and consequent weakening of bone density (Fig. 47, Fig. 48).

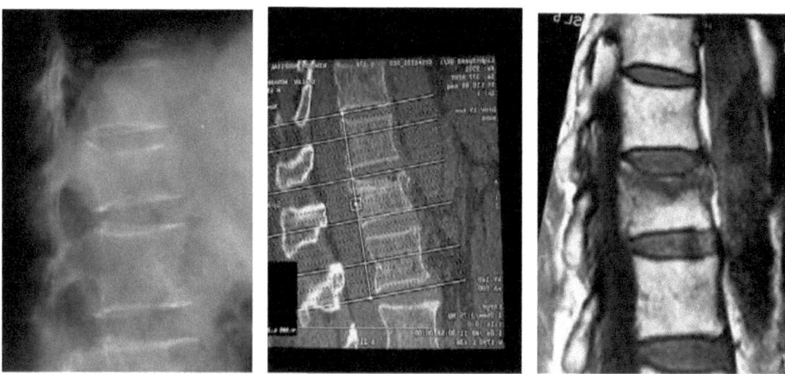

Figure 47: Imaging of spinal compression fracture on radiographs, CT and MRI in the acute period.

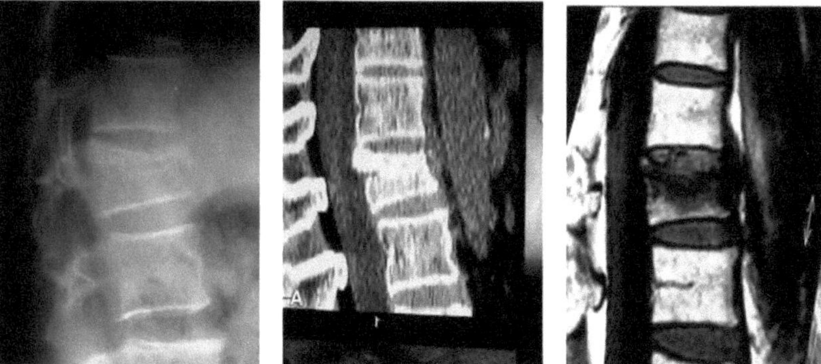

Figure 48: Image of the same spine 2.5 months after injury.

The degree of compression has increased (radiographs and CT scan). MRI shows hyperintense signal spreading to the entire vertebral body.

First of all, the compression of the spinal cord by bony structures, the degree of deformity and narrowing of the spinal canal, and the deformity and degree of narrowing and deformation of the dural sac are revealed. (Figure 49).

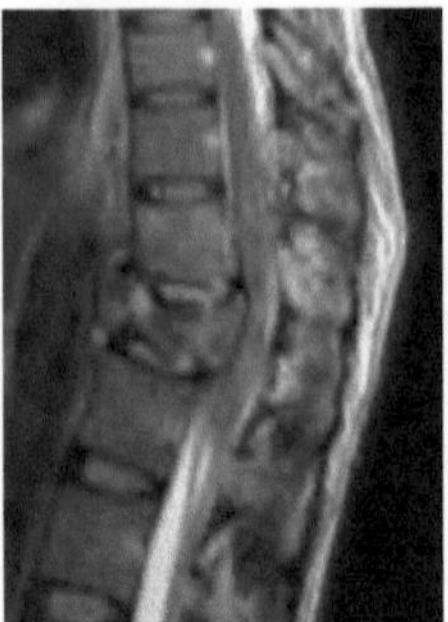

Figure 49. MRI of the lumbar spine. Compression of the spinal cord by bony structures, deformation and narrowing of the spinal canal and dural sac.

In addition to dural sac deformity and narrowing, MRI may also show changes in the spinal cord. An area of hyperintense signal in the spinal cord may be seen at the level of the injury, which may indicate spinal cord contusion or hematomyelia (Figure 50).

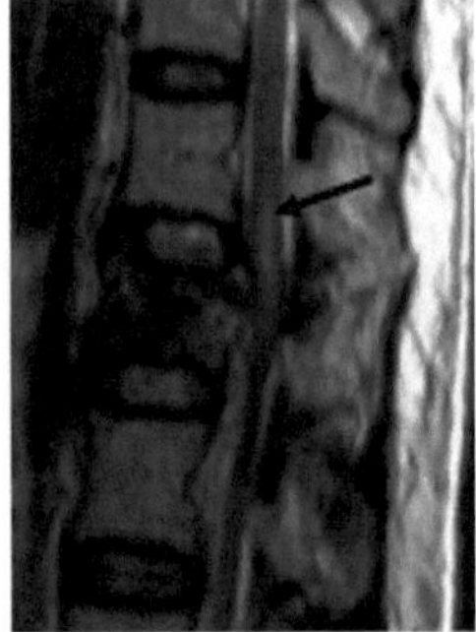

Figure 50. MRI of the lumbar region. An area of hyperintense signal is seen in the spinal cord

In the absence of bony lesions on radiographs and CT scans but a clinical picture of spinal cord injury, MRI may show a hyperintense signal in the posterior ligamentous complex, which would indicate a loss of posterior ligamentous complex integrity (Figure 51).

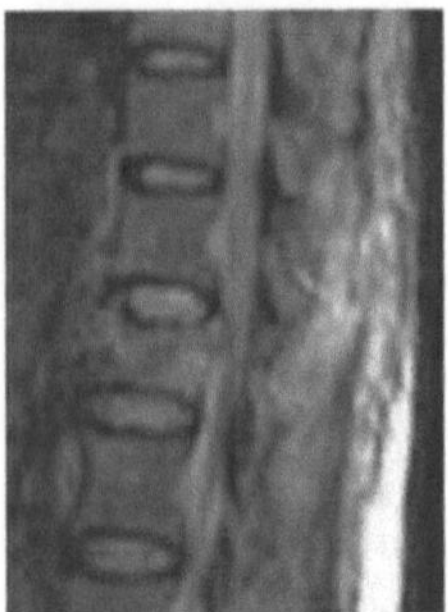

Figure 51. MRI of the lumbar spine. Hyperintense signal in the posterior ligamentous complex

In the case of vertebral dislocations in the form of dislocations or subluxations, a significant narrowing of the spinal cord cross-section and its compression by protruding bone fragments can be detected. Hyperintense signal of the spinal cord can be seen not only at the level of the lesion, but also at the level of superior and inferior segments. Hyperintense signal may also be present in the bodies of apparently intact vertebrae, which may indicate moderate vertebral damage without disruption of the bony structure. (Figure 52).

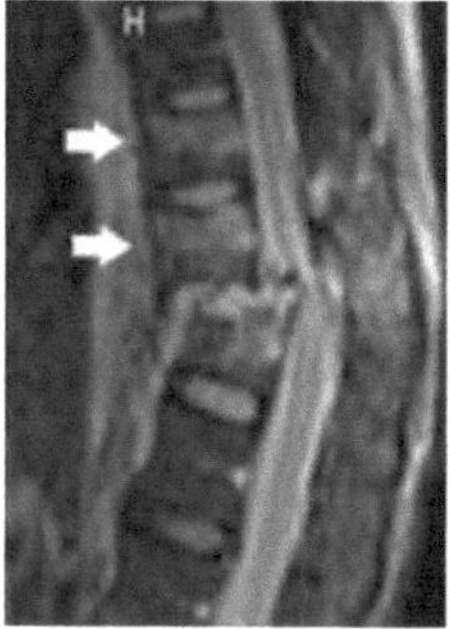

Figure 52. MRI of the lumbar spine. Hyperintense signal of the spinal cord above the level of spinal cord injury and brain compression. Hyperintense signal in the bodies of the overlying vertebrae (indicated by arrows).

A transverse spinal cord injury visible on MRI indicates a severe injury with no chance of restoring spinal cord function. Deformity correction and spinal stabilization is possible and necessary for early social rehabilitation of the patient (Figure 53).

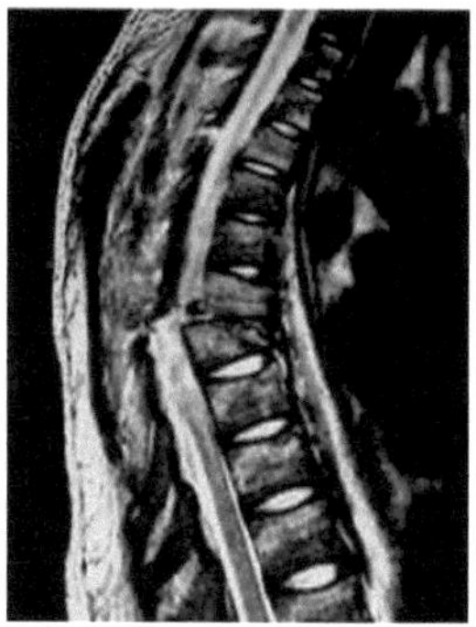

Figure 53. MRI of a fracture-dislocation of the Th6 vertebra. Complete transverse spinal cord injury is seen.

MRI typically captures a region of the spine that spans multiple vertebral segments. When analyzing MRI, in addition to changes at the level under investigation, traumatic changes can be detected in distant segments. In such cases, a multilevel injury is involved (Figure 54).

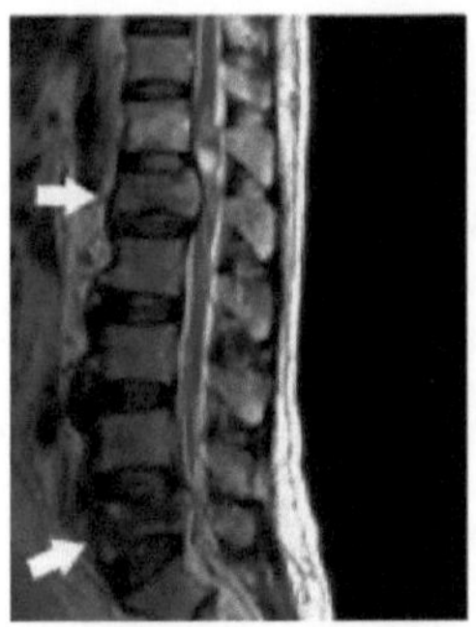

Figure 54. MRI of the lumbar spine. Multilevel injury. In addition to damage to the vertebral bodies, an isolated hyperintense focus in the spinal cord is seen.

Below are illustrations of the correspondence of vertebral lesions on radiographs and CT scans to the AO/ASIF classification.

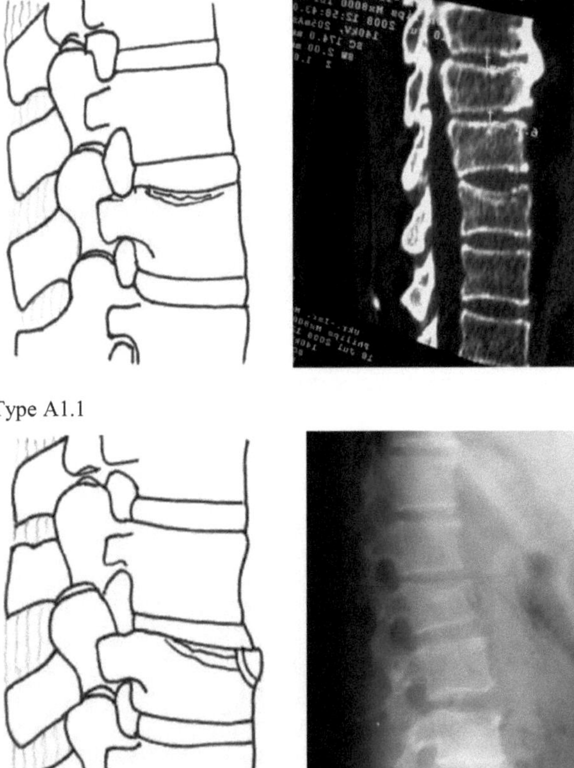

Type A1.1

Type A1.2

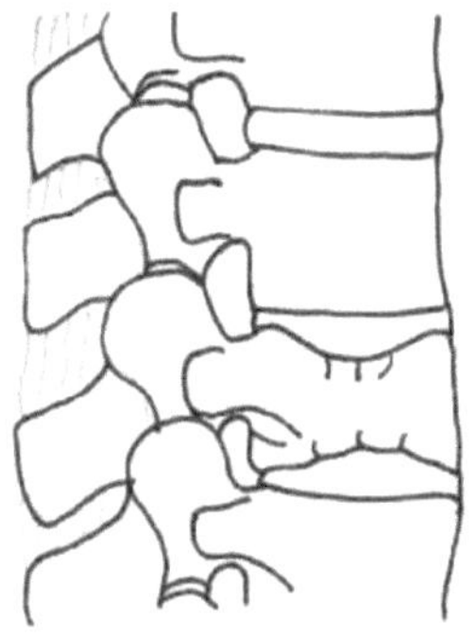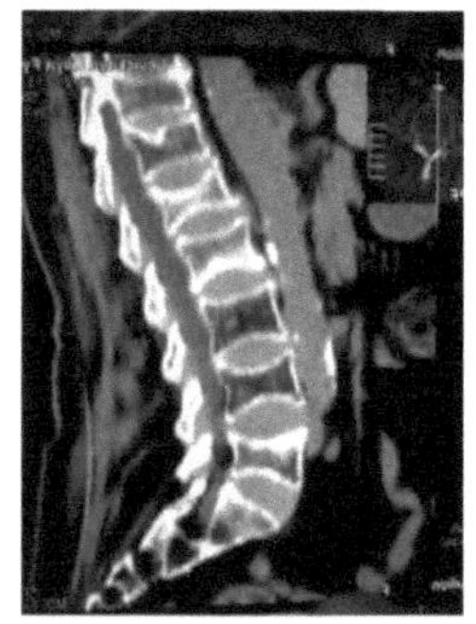

Type A1.3

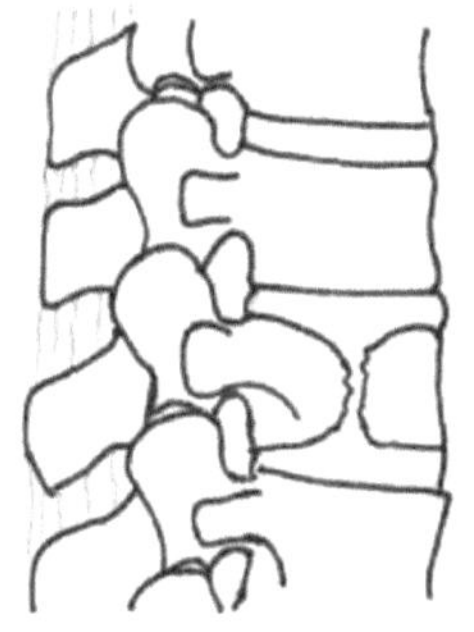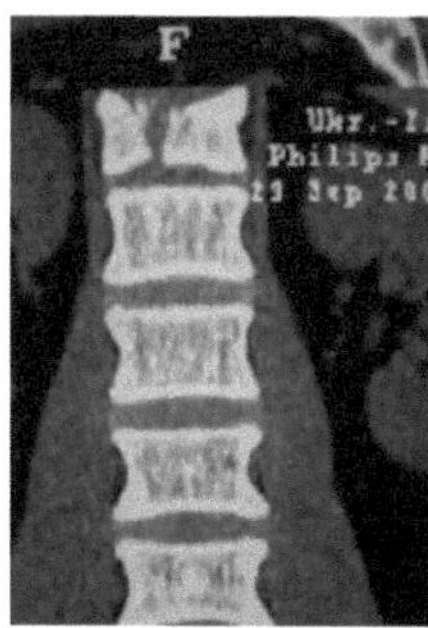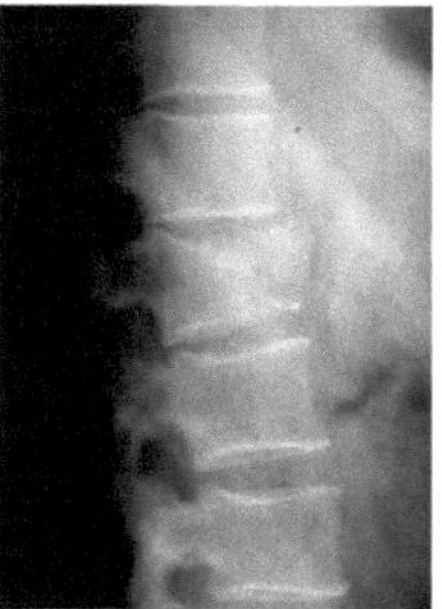

Type A2.1 - Type A2.2

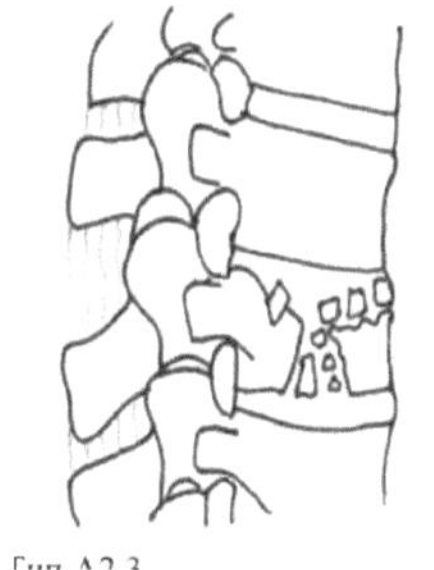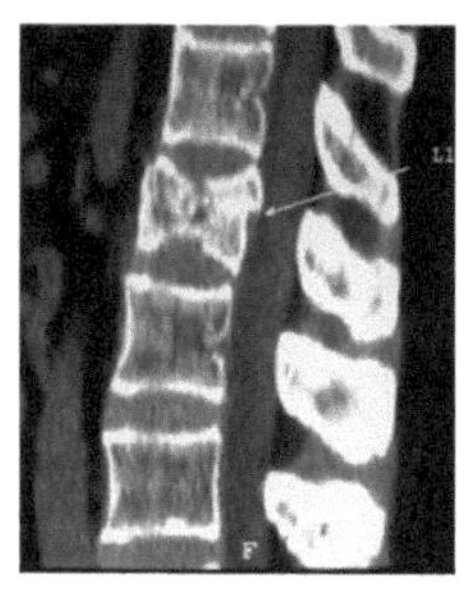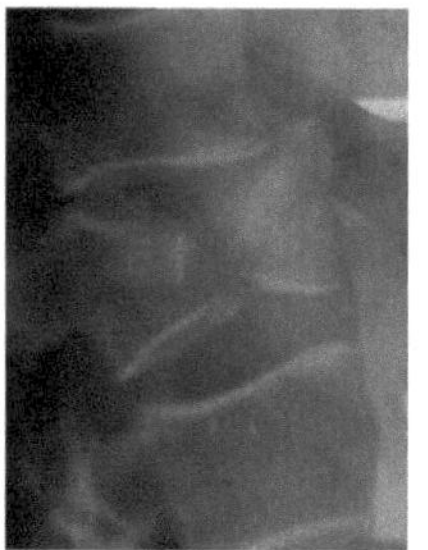

Type A2.3.

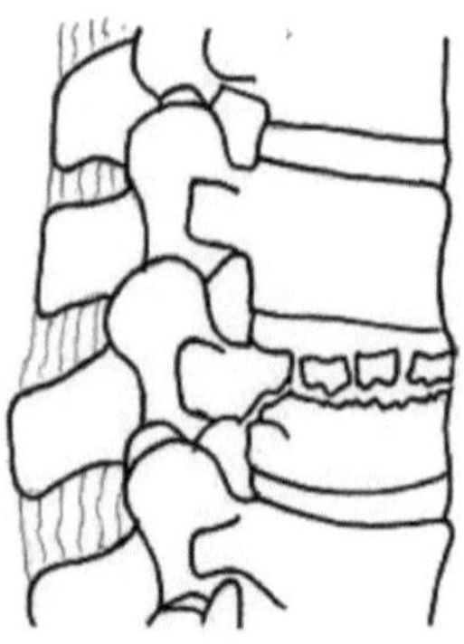 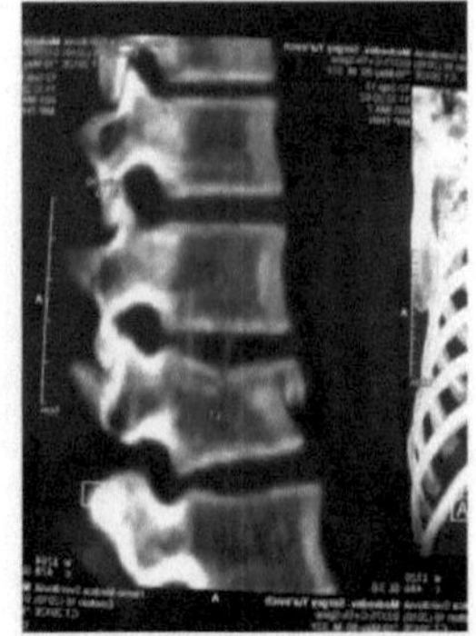

Type A3.1.

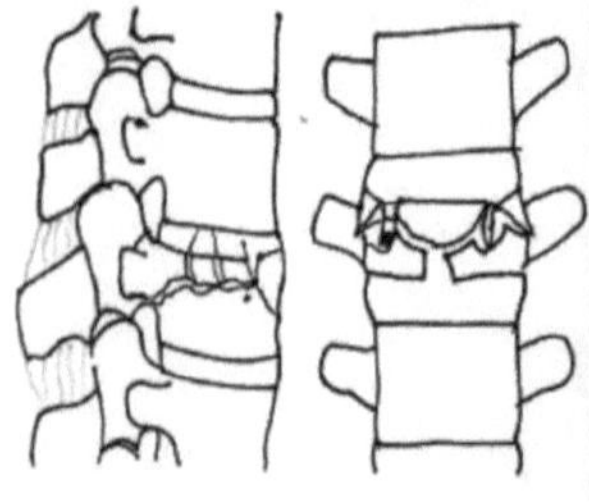 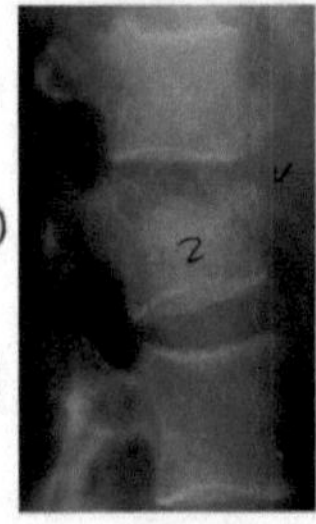 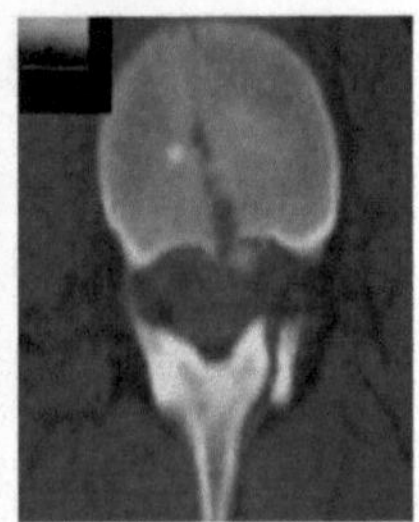

Type A3.2.

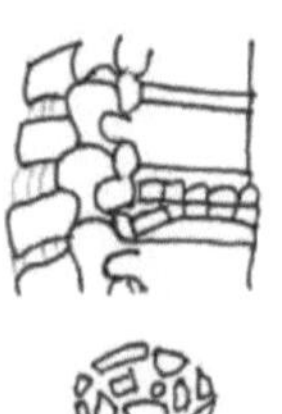
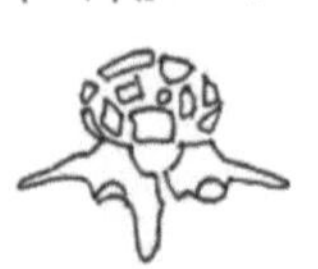 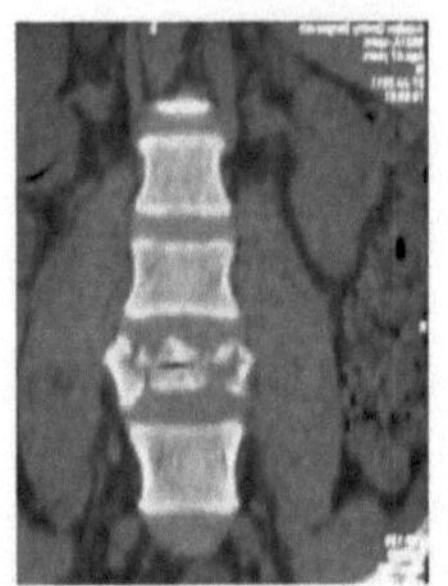 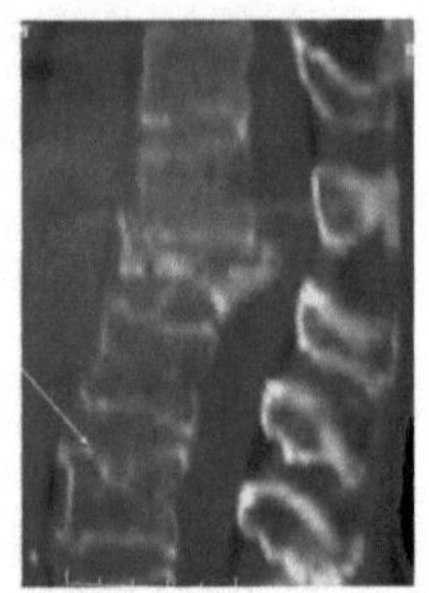

Type A 3.3

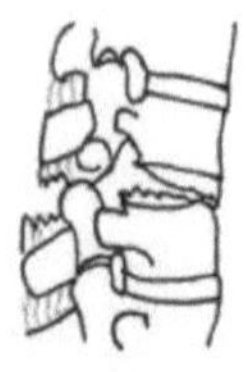 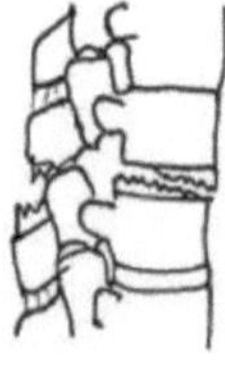 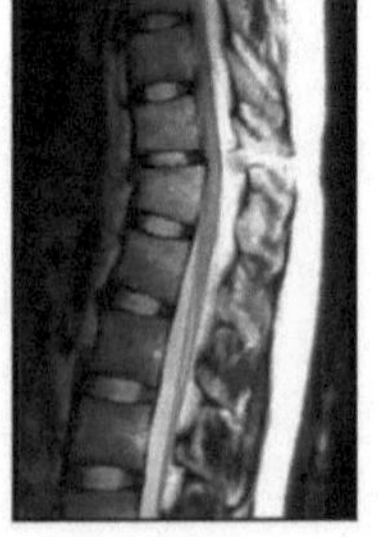 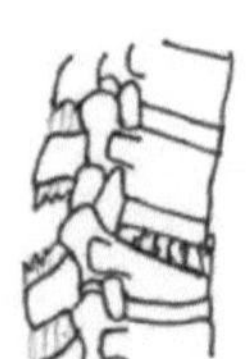 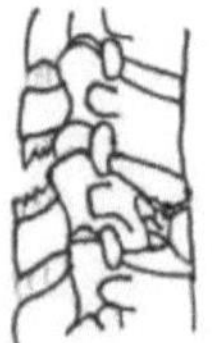

Type B 1.1 to B 1.2.

Type B 2.1. Type B 2.2. Type B 2.3.

Type C 1.1.

Type C 1.2.

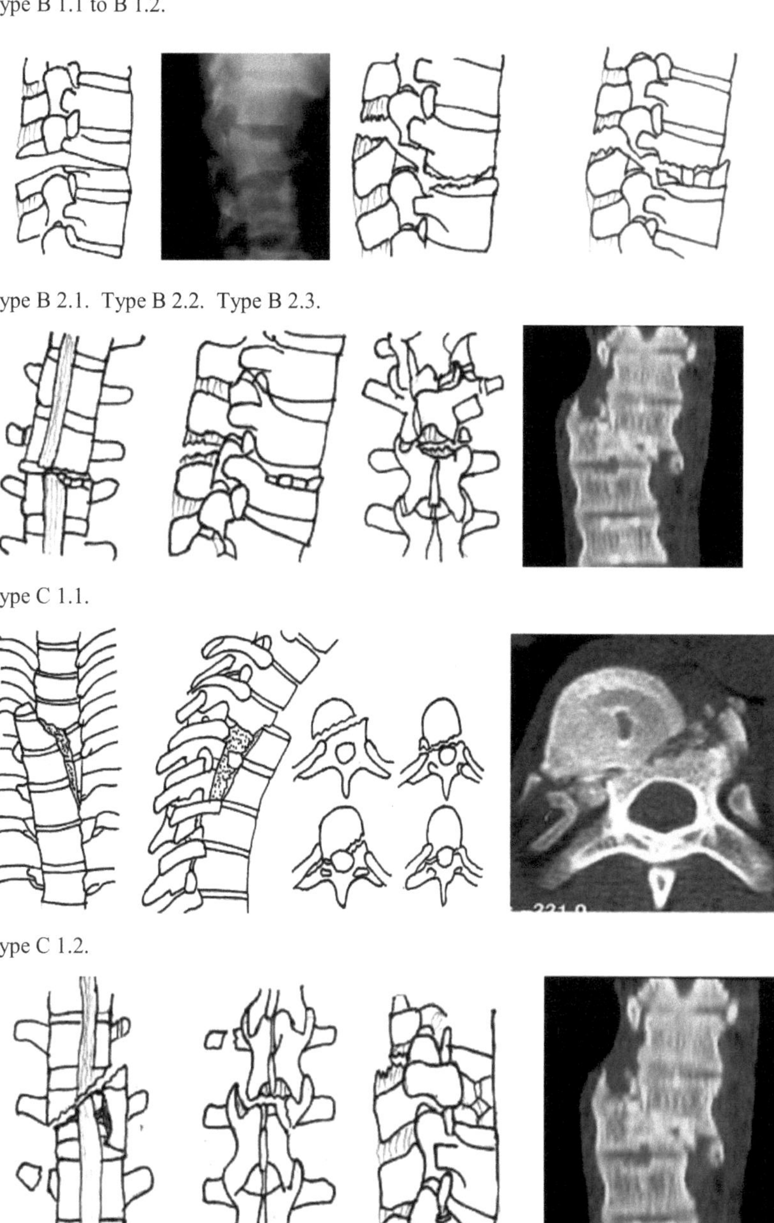

Type C 1.3.

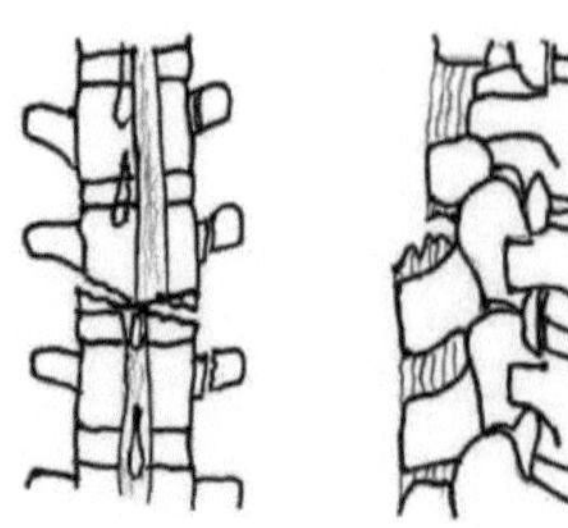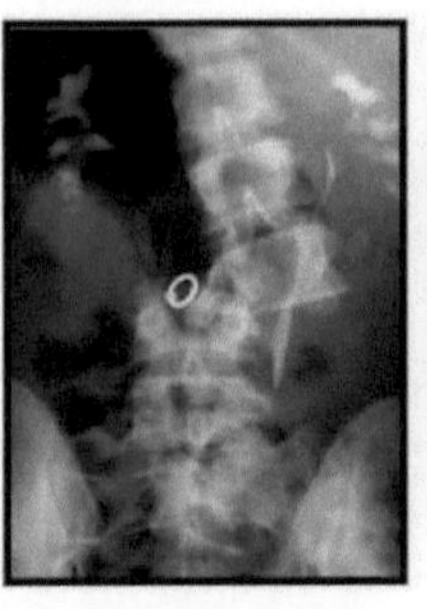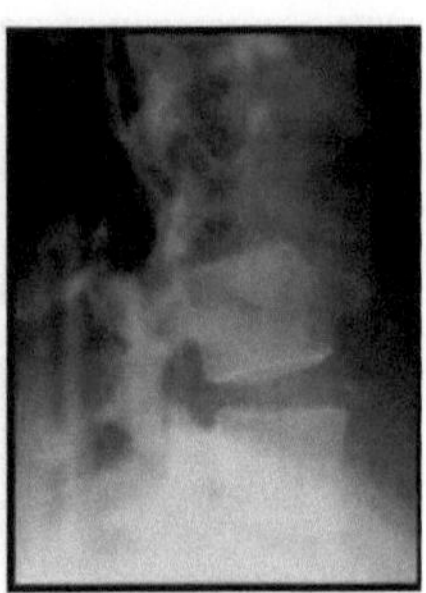

Type C 2.1.

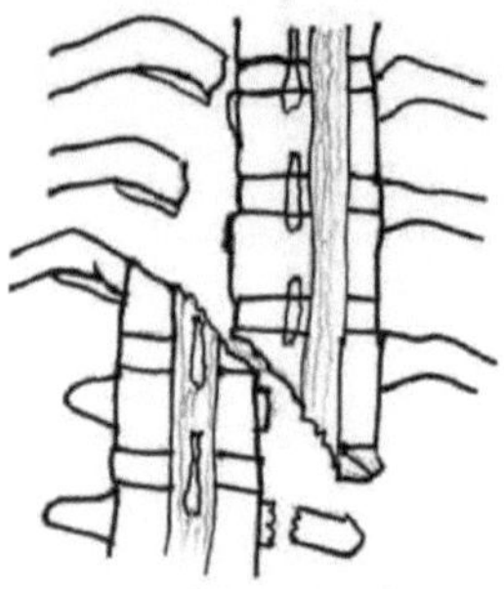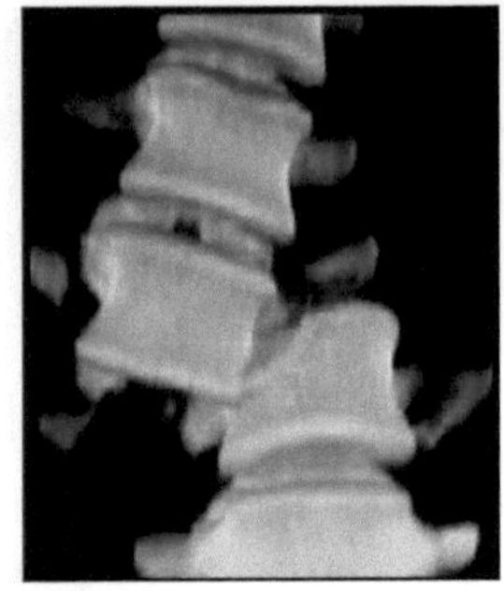

Type C 3.2.

Injuries to the sacrum

The sacrum, as an anatomical structure, is a section of the vertebral column and at the same time is an integral part of the pelvis. Fractures of the sacrum are rare and more than 90% are associated with pelvic fractures. In the structure of spinal fractures, they account for 5-10% of all spinal fractures

Lumbosacral segment injuries are always the result of high energy injuries and are often one component of unstable pelvic fractures or polytrauma.

Lumbosacral injuries may be missed during the initial imaging. Radiographs taken in the acute care setting often do not provide adequate information. On R-gram, 60% of sacral fractures are initially undiagnosed. (Lafollette, Levine, and McNiesh) An indirect sign such as an L5 transverse process fracture is often a sign of a more serious injury in the lumbosacral segment.

Due to the layering of large bone masses on top of each other, radiographs of the sacrum in the standard straight view (pelvic radiograph) may not reveal damage in its upper segments. In some cases, pelvic radiography in the oblique view (Outlet view) can provide additional information in such situations (Fig. 55).

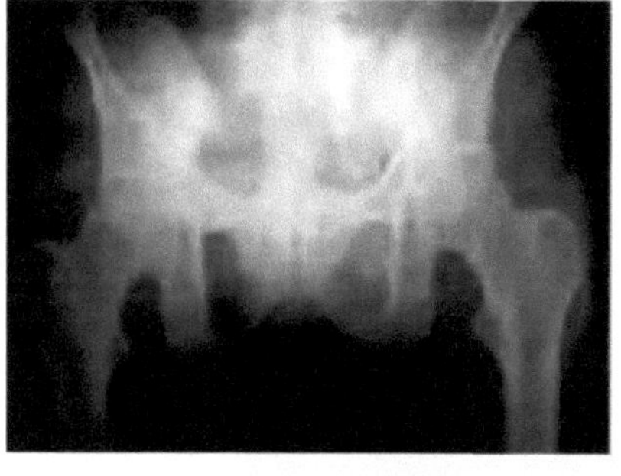

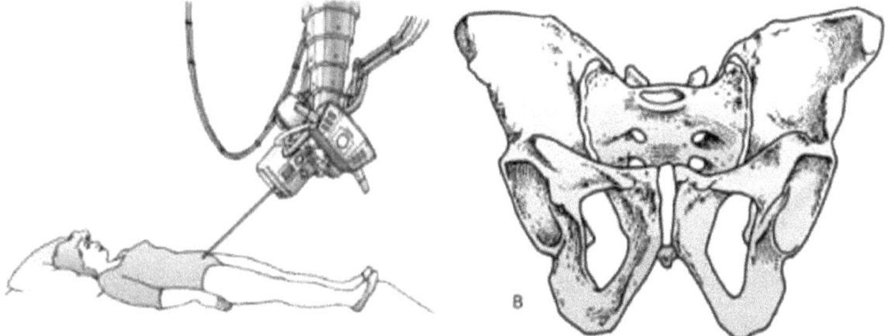

Figure 55. Oblique projection - for anterior half-ring (Outlet view)-CHU3y upwards

In terms of the nature of the injury, sacral fractures can be transverse (Figure 57), longitudinal unilateral and bilateral, and splinter fractures (Figure 59).

Vertical fractures of the sacrum are classified by Denis into 3 zones based on localization of the fracture line: lateral mass zone, sacral foramen zone, and sacral (spinal) zone (Figure 56).

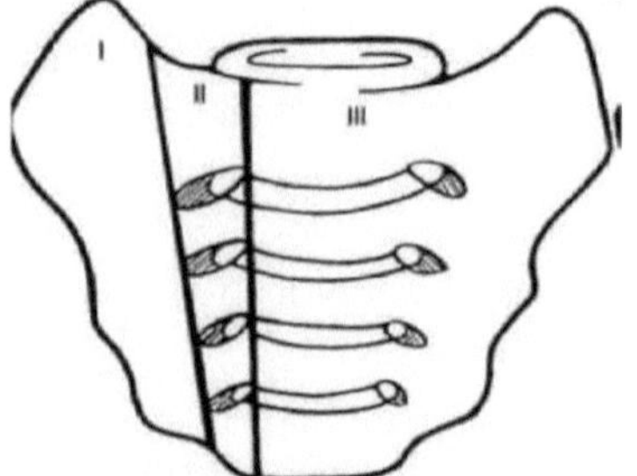

Fig.56. Denis classification of pelvic fracture: 3 zones of injury: - zone I, lateral masses (wings) of the sacrum; - zone II, sacral foramen region; - zone III, spinal canal (Denis F, Davis S, Comfort T: Clin Orthop 227:67, 1988)

The vertical fractures may be partial, involving only a portion of the lateral masses of the upper sacral vertebrae, or complete, passing through the entire sacrum (Figs. 58, 59).

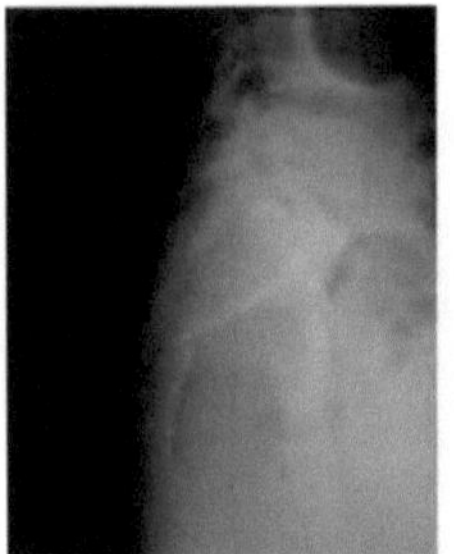
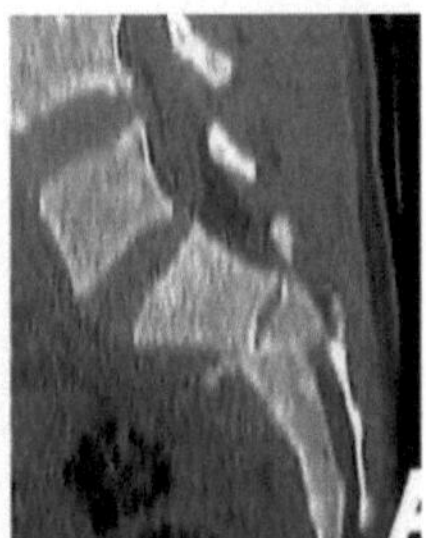

Figure 57. Stable fractures - transverse fractures of the sacrum (complicated and uncomplicated)

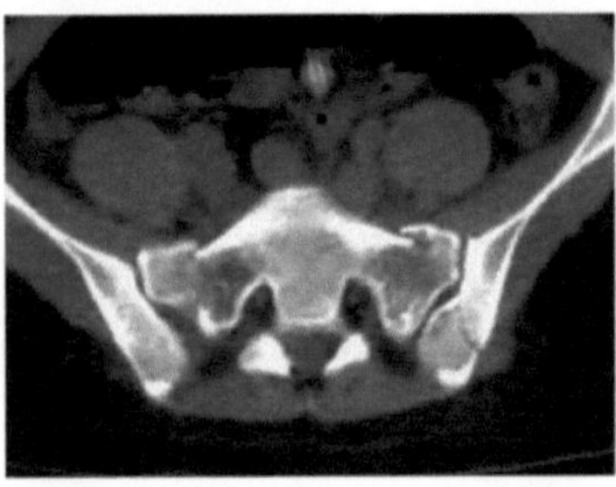
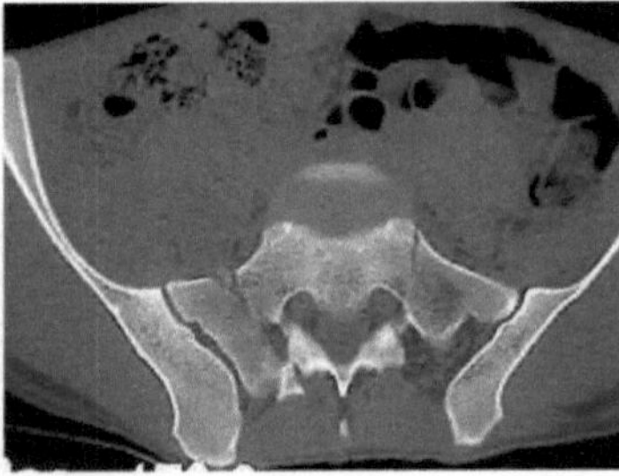

Figure 58. Relatively stable sacral fractures (partial vertical)

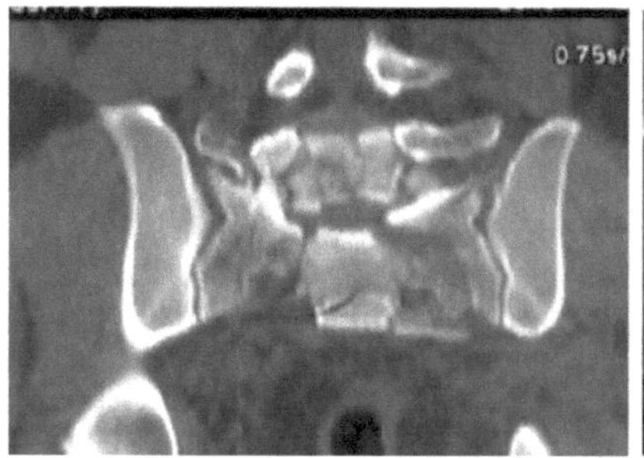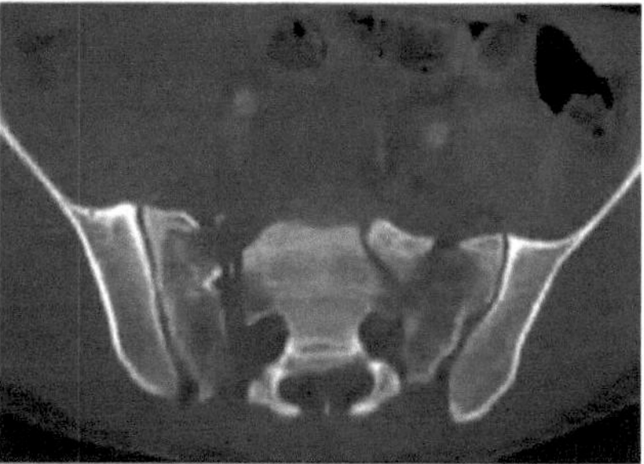

Figure 59. Vertical bilateral fracture of the sacrum in combination with a fragmentary unstable fracture of the L5 vertebrae

Literature

1. Korzh N.A. Instability of the cervical spine: Dissertation ...doctor of medical sciences, - Kharkov, 1985.- 433 p.

2. Polishchuk N.E., Korzh N.A.. , Fishchenko V.Ya. Spinal cord and spinal cord injuries (mechanisms, clinic, diagnostics, treatment).Kiev.-2001.-387 p.

3. Radchenko V.A., Korzh N.A. Practicum on stabilization of thoracic and lumbar vertebral divisions.-"Prapor" Kharkov 2004.- 156 p.

4. Selivanov V.P., Nikitin M.N. Diagnosis and treatment of cervical vertebrae dislocations (edited by L.G. Shkolnikov).-M.:Medicine,1971.-328 pp.

5. An H.S., Angthong C., Wunnasinthop S., Sanpakit S. Complex lumbosacral fracturedislocation with pelvic ring disruption and vertical shear sacral fracture: a case report of late presentation and review of the literature // Turkish Journal of Trauma & Emergency Surgery. 2010;16 (6): P. 561-566.

6. Hashimoto T., Kaneda K., Abumi K.. Relationship between traumatic spinal canal stenosis and neurologic deficits in thoracolumbar burst fractures // Spine (Phila. Pa. 1976). - 1988. - Vol. 13, № 11. - P. 1268-1272.

7. Max Aebi, Vincent Arlet, John K Webb. AO Spine Manual Principles and Techniques. // Thieme New York, 2007.-663 p.

8. Mouhsine E., Wettstein M., Schizas C. et al. Modified triangular posterior osteosynthesis of unstable sacrum fracture // Eur. Spine J. 2006 June; 15(6): P. 857-863.

9. Nork S.E., Jones C.B., Harding S.P. et al. Percutaneous stabilization of U-shaped sacral fractures using iliosacral screws : technique and early results // J. Orthop. Orthop. Trauma. 2001; 15: P. 238-246.

10. Rasmussen P.A., Rabin M.H., Mann D.C., Perl J.R., Lorenz M.A., Vrbos Reduced L.A. Transverse spinal area secondary to burst fractures: is there a relationship to neurologic injury? // J. Neurotrauma. Neurotrauma. - 1994. - Vol. 11, № 6. - P. 711-720.

11. Sedat J., Chau Y., Razafidratsiva C. et al. One-Stage Percutaneous Treatment in a Patient with Pelvic and Vertebral Compression Fractures // Cardiovasc. Intervent Radiol. (2010) 33: P. 219-222.

12. Simpson M.I. Surgery of the cervical spine //Martiw Dunitz Ltd.,- 1994.- 432 p.White A.A., Panjabi M.M. Clinical Biomechanics of the Spine.- New York: Lippincott.- 1990.

13. Tsirikos A.I., Saifuddin, M.H.. Noordeen et al. Traumatic lumbosacral dislocation: report of two cases // Spine (Phila Pa 1976) 2004; 29: E164-168.

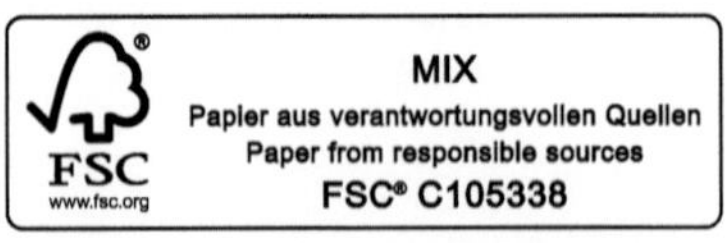

Printed by Books on Demand GmbH, Norderstedt / Germany